"Even if you've never lifted a kettlebell, you'll be fascinated by Madden's view of the challenges and psychology behind the phenomenon."               —*Self*

"Surprisingly personal and compelling . . . Madden's epiphanies are genuine, and well rendered. . . . He may be subpar as an athlete. He's far, far above that as a writer."
                                              —*Sports Illustrated*

"Madden's entertaining and inspiring fitness memoir is ultimately about life, love, and so much more."
                                              —*Reader's Digest*

"As a slovenly layman outsider, I'd often found CrossFit intimidating and cultish. But Stephen Madden's engaging, open, and funny book about how it changed his life—but kept him resolutely who he is—did away with all that: He finds the human side of the sport, the activity, and the community. A perfect introduction to a worldview that can change yours."
        —Will Leitch, founder of Deadspin.com, contributing editor for *New York* magazine, and author of *God Save the Fan* and *Are We Winning?*

"This is a great book about getting fit and what it takes to endure the hell of diet, muscle-ups, and nausea of Cross-Fit training. But unexpectedly, it is about much more. A book that seemed to be about tough-minded, solitary self-improvement for masters-of-the-universe types turned out to be a story about sharing, community, and love. That's right! So, while you couldn't pay me to do all the burpees, dead lifts, and muscle-ups that Madden endures, I will pay for copies of this book to hand around to my friends. Turns out in sports, according to Madden, winning isn't everything: It still matters how you play the game."

—Alex Gibney, Academy Award–winning writer and director of *Taxi to the Dark Side*

"Too few people are able or willing to plumb the depths of what sport, suffering, and physical challenge really mean to us. Here Stephen Madden gets far beyond any simple notions of winning, losing, going faster, or getting stronger, and goes to a place where triumph and failure become primal elements of life. What's as impressive is that he comes back with such a well-told tale."

—Bill Strickland, editor-in-chief of *Bicycling* magazine and author of *Ten Points*

"The numerous workout anecdotes will entertain the CrossFit faithful, but Madden's well-written personal narrative may appeal to a more general fitness audience."

—*Booklist*

# EMBRACE THE SUCK

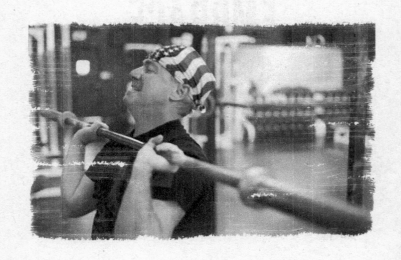

# EMBRACE THE SUCK

## What I Learned at the Box About Hard Work, (Very) Sore Muscles, and Burpees Before Sunrise

## STEPHEN MADDEN

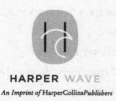

HARPER WAVE

*An Imprint of HarperCollinsPublishers*

HarperCollins
PUBLISHERS
*Since 1817*

A hardcover edition of this book was published in 2014 by Harper Wave, an imprint of HarperCollins Publishers.

HarperCollins books may be purchased for educational, business, or sales promotional use. For information, please e-mail the Special Markets Department at SPsales@harpercollins.com.

FIRST HARPER WAVE PAPERBACK EDITION PUBLISHED 2017.

*Designed by William Ruoto*

Frontispiece courtesy of Mickey Brueckner

Library of Congress Cataloging-in-Publication Data has been applied for.

ISBN 978-0-06-225787-1 (pbk.)

HB 01.29.2020

For Winifred Shannon Madden and Anne Thompson,
who show me every day that love, strength, and
patience are all the same thing.

We choose to go to the moon in this decade and do the other things, not because they are easy, but because they are hard.

—John F. Kennedy, September 12, 1962

# Contents

Contents

# Introduction

On a warm, overcast Saturday morning in July 2012, I stood, shirtless and barefoot, in the deep, dry sand of the beach in Avon, New Jersey, a 25-pound Tyvek bag of sand draped across my shoulders and neck in the same manner some other beachgoers that day carried plush towels. I was among two hundred people, most of them half my age, overwhelmingly male, astonishingly fit, breathtakingly tattooed—many with "Semper Fi" and "FTW," a veteran's mark of honor. Their mere presence made me self-conscious of the gray tufts of hair on my chest and the spare tire of fat around my waist. That the spare now resembled more of a bicycle tire and less of the tractor tire it had a few years ago was beside the point. Just a couple of hours earlier, safe in my suburban home, I had caught a glimpse of myself in a mirror and thought, "Hey, hotshot. Not looking too bad for a forty-eight-year-old. All those early morning workouts are paying off. Gonna look great at the pool club this afternoon." It was one of the first times in my life that I looked in the mirror and truly liked the body I saw. But now, among the hyperfit, I was reduced once again to being the fat kid on the playground, a twelve-year-old who wants desperately to play but has trouble getting in the game. And when he does, is just not that good.

I was about to dive into the deep end of the sport of fitness as a participant in the second annual Warrior Challenge, a competition designed to test the overall fitness of its contestants with feats of endurance, strength, and speed.

And I was about to get my ass kicked.

After the presentation of the colors and the singing of the national anthem, an air horn blared and the first event, the sandbag carry, was off. We set off down the beach along a row of orange barrels that stretched for a quarter of a mile. We went at various paces, some at what sure looked to me like a dead sprint, some at a trot, me at a jog. That jog would last for four hundred yards, to the turnaround point, where my ragged breath and aching legs suggested I take it down a notch, to a brisk walk. That lasted another two hundred yards, until the walk became much less brisk. On the other side of the row of barrels, the leaders were running the second of their two laps, but without sandbags. When I reached the point where I had started, a far-too-enthusiastic volunteer told me I could ditch the bag and "Really go for it!" It sounded like a good idea, but my legs, my lungs, and, increasingly, my mind would not comply. So I took up a strategy I had come to employ the last few years: I would chip away. I would run as best as I could from one barrel to the next, then walk to the next one. It was agonizing, and agonizingly slow, as I was at first lapped by the race leaders and then passed by people who, in my alternate reality, had no right passing me. Women with cellulite in bike shorts. A man, much older than I, who smiled at me and said, "Not bad for an old guy, huh?"

When I finished, finally, mercifully, that mile in the sand, I doubled over at the knees and watched my dripping sweat form miniature concretions on the sand underneath me. Luke, my twelve-year-old son, approached cautiously. I had seen him watching over the top of a book while I struggled by with the sandbag.

"Hi," he said.

"Hi," I gasped. "What did you think of that?"

"I thought this was a race."

"It is."

"You didn't look like you were racing. You didn't look like you were trying very hard. Some of those other guys were putting out"—a phrase we often used to mean working hard—"and you weren't."

Here I was, my legs jelled and my lungs and breakfast both about to come out of my throat, and my own seed was telling me I wasn't working hard enough.

The truth is, I didn't need him to tell me that. I have been telling myself that nearly every day of my life, and especially since I first started the particular form of training called CrossFit. Those who follow CrossFit, by doing the Workouts of the Day (WODing), are known for the fervor they feel for the program, and the true belief they place in its tenets. The results are undeniable. Those who strictly follow the exercise program and its attendant dietary regimens like the Zone or Paleo diets, develop amazing physiques marked by the broad chests and backs, skinny waists, and huge quads of the actors who performed in the film *300*, all of whom were whipped into shape by trainers with a background in CrossFit. The idea is to create athletes who can do lots of different movements quickly, and for a long time. In other words, to be prepared for anything the physical world might throw at you.

All you have to do is lift more weight than you thought you could more times than you thought human in as short a period of time as possible. Or perform gymnastics moves, plyometrics, and calisthenics in agonizing combinations designed to identify and rub out your weaknesses. Or impale yourself on a rowing machine or on runs ranging anywhere from ten yards to ten kilometers. Most CrossFit workouts last less than twenty minutes and involve some combination of the above. The trick, however, is going as fast as you possibly can. To complete As Many Rounds as Possible (AMRAP) in a prescribed period of time, or to do a set number of repetitions as quickly as possible. Yes, CrossFit hurts. It's supposed to hurt. If it didn't, the thinking goes, then everybody would do it. The fact that it seemed like everybody *was* doing it didn't dawn on me for a while: there are more than ten thousand CrossFit gyms around the world, and more than two million people count themselves among the faithful.

I first learned about CrossFit in, of all places, a 2005 article in the Thursday Style section of the *New York Times*. I, like a lot of people who count that piece as their point of entry, was intrigued by the description of a sport with its own mascots: Pukie the Clown, who often visited athletes, and Uncle Rhabdo, short for rhabdomyolosis, a dangerous condition caused by muscle breakdown from intense exercise. Not that I wanted to puke or end up on dialysis, but I did want to learn more.

At the time, I was the editor in chief of *Bicycling* magazine, and in excellent cycling shape. The article intrigued me, however, because it was published at a point in the year when I was looking for something to do in the winter as an adjunct to my indoor cycling training. I spent some time on crossfit.com, which was rich with illustrative video files that demonstrated the exercises. And then, in a gym, I tried a workout. It was utterly impossible for me to finish. Here I was, capable of riding a bike 100 miles over the French Alps, but incapable of lifting 100 pounds over my head, or doing 25 push-ups, or completing three 800-meter runs.

So I tried it again. And again. And again. I made some headway, just enough to keep me coming back. When spring rolled around, I got back on my bike but kept doing a couple of CrossFit routines each week with some rudimentary weights and mats in my garage. My cyclist's sunken chest started to grow, and my shoulders, rounded by endless miles hunched over handlebars, squared off. I attended a weekend-long class, a "cert," designed to teach me the fundamentals of the program. I went, I took notes, I participated with the other students, came in near to dead last in the sample workouts. But I didn't care. I loved it, even if it left me gasping for air and prostrate at the end of each workout, and unable to climb the thirty-two steps from Penn Station to Eighth Avenue the next day.

But I wasn't fully committed. I still ate whatever I wanted, whenever I wanted. I rode my bike and I swam, and I dabbled in CrossFit. I could now complete workouts that would leave most men my age injured or crying or both. And I could pretty much do whatever activity I wanted—swim a mile, ride seventy-five, hike all day—without hurting myself. But I couldn't complete all the CrossFit exercises as prescribed. I couldn't, as CrossFitters say, Rx. Muscle-ups eluded me. My pull-ups were woeful. And while I had learned the techniques of the Olympic weight moves, the amount of weight I could handle was, on a good day, equal to the women's standard. The spare tire was stubbornly still inflated.

I was fit. But not truly CrossFit.

And I showed it that day in Avon. After the run, we lined up in front of chin-up bars to see how many "strict" pull-ups we could do. A strict pull-up is just that. You hang, arms fully extended, from the bar, with your palms facing away from you. You keep your legs and hips still, and you use all your upper body strength to get your chin over the bar. You then drop back down, all the way down, hanging, and do it again, as many times as you can. The guys ahead of me were doing 11, 17, 23.

I did three.

I fared better at the burpees, that old gym class chestnut of throwing yourself flat out on the ground, then hopping back up as quickly as you can, jumping up and clapping your hands over your head. I was able to do 32, again in deep sand, in the prescribed two minutes. Respectable. After a little rest, I squeezed out 52 sit-ups in two minutes. That was about average.

And that was that. Run in the sand. Do some calisthenics. I finished close to the bottom of all male competitors; there were a few guys in my age group slower and weaker than me. But not many. I took some solace in that fact that not many men in their forties had decided to do this.

By nightfall, I'd be unable to do much of anything but lie on the couch and wonder why, after all this training, I sucked as badly as I did. The thought was compounded by another question: Why did I want to pursue something I sucked at while making myself so goddamn sore? What was it about this stuff?

I thought back to a moment from earlier in the day, before the competition started. I had checked in, pinned my race number to my shorts, and started to warm up, moving my arms and legs in slow, ever-expanding circles to loosen the muscles, get the blood moving and slowly raise my heart rate. It was a routine I had followed for years before events like the Warrior Challenge. Before swimming across Tampa Bay or Chesapeake Bay or along the shores of St. John in the U.S. Virgin Islands. Before the Empire State Games swimming championship. Before the Boston and New York City marathons. Before climbing Mount Rainier in summer or in the White Mountains in winter. Before every rinky-dink 5K I ever ran. Before track meets, bike races, indoor rowing competitions, cross-country ski races, snowshoe races, triathlons, biathlons, duathlons, kayak races, mountain bike races. All of them, with me warming up the same way. Slow circles, slow, easy motions. Warming up, getting ready.

And wondering, before each and every one of them, just what the fuck was I doing here? What was I trying to prove, and to whom was I trying to prove it? What was I after and could it even be found in something as ultimately trivial as, say, a pull-up contest? Some people invest their self-worth in the quality of their relationships or their work, or perhaps with their relationship to higher powers. For some reason, I had decided that meaning lay in how many burpees I could do in the sand or how fast I could swim a mile.

These thoughts had been with me as long as I could remember, and I'd never been able to answer the question or banish the doubt. They didn't prevent me from competing, and certainly not from training, which from junior high through college and then again since age twenty-six had been as much a part of my daily routine as brushing my teeth, reading the sports section, or drinking coffee. The questions often came up before workouts, too. They asked themselves loudest before races, but they nagged every day. If the unexamined life was not worth living, then I was in need of a checkout. Because I couldn't answer questions that had haunted me so long I couldn't remember when they first raised their hands. And I was sick to fucking death of them nagging me.

I needed to answer the questions. It was time. They

had been with me long enough. I knew that deep down, this had very little to do with exercise. I was hoping to find some other, larger truth in all this. I was nearing fifty, and I was feeling weird. I had a job. I had my health. I had a family and friends and people who loved me. But I often felt like a spectator in my own life, overwhelmed by responsibilities and the sense that at any moment I would fail, that I was still not doing exactly what I wanted to be doing, because I still didn't know what that was.

I had stumbled across a saying that soldiers and marines in Iraq and Afghanistan had been using to describe a coping mechanism that got them through their deployments: Embrace the Suck. Yeah, it sucks here. But here you are. And wishing it didn't suck wasn't going to make it any less sucky, so make the best of it by embracing it and seeing what lessons can be learned from it.

There was a lesson in there for my whole life. I had just left a comfortable job I had held for eleven years, and traded an understanding, supportive boss for four demanding new ones in the form of the board of directors of the Internet start-up I was running. I was telling prospective employees that the next couple of years would be uncomfortable and could, quite possibly, suck.

That was it: I wasn't embracing the suck. Rather than leaning in to the pain of a workout or a race to hear what it was telling me, I was avoiding it and letting my mind wander so that I wasn't getting the whole message. As a result,

I wasn't getting the whole benefit. Sure, my muscles got sore and I gasped for breath. But I had the strong sense I was missing something. My wife, Anne Thompson, is one of the most ferociously competitive people I know. She's capable of impaling herself fully on a workout, jumping onto it without fear. She never says a workout was good, rather that it sucked, which is her way of saying that it was good. She's far more interested in the benefit of the workout rather than the process. In that respect she is my opposite. She regularly looks at me after a workout and shakes her head. "You could have gone way harder," she says.

That would change. Instead of saying, "Wow, man, these hundred burpees are just about the worst thing ever besides a kick in the nuts," and thinking about how awful the next twenty minutes were going to be, I'd lean in. I'd listen to it. There was an answer in there somewhere. I'd hear that what the soreness and lactic acid was telling me, what weaknesses it was pointing out, what I needed to work on. And who knows? If it was going well, maybe I'd be able to say, "Wow! those burpees really do make every muscle in your body stronger!" When the bile rose in my throat, I'd taste it to see what message it carried (besides the importance of never, ever drinking coffee before a WOD).

The path to the answer to the question "Why the fuck am I doing this?" was clear.

I needed to embrace the suck.

# EMBRACE THE SUCK

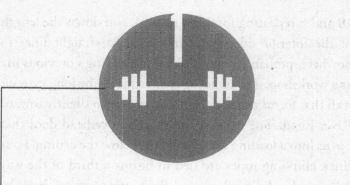

# The WOD

I have studied the ceiling of the Annex, an athletic training facility in the small industrial area of the otherwise leafy suburb of Chatham, New Jersey, as if it were the Sistine Chapel. It is a wonder of textured white, thanks to the corrugated panels that form its body, with rafters running the length of the building, and beams spanning the width. Heating ducts, the pieces numbered 1–25 (with

18 and 5 repeating for some reason), run down the length of the interior side, and wires hang in straight lines to nowhere, probably remnants of the building's previous life as a workshop. The building is not square: the long exterior wall that forms the back slants away ever so slightly toward River Road. The runners for a sliding overhead door that opens into a loading dock hang just below the ceiling. Four thick climbing ropes are tied to beams a third of the way in from the sliding door, and the heating system, built by Reznor, a company founded by an ancestor of Nine Inch Nails frontman Trent Reznor, hangs near a vent to the outside. Speakers dangle from two locations and pour out a never-ending stream of high-beats-per-minute music that ranges from rap to classic rock to house, depending on who's controlling Pandora on the iPhone plugged into the sound system.

I'd never paid much attention to a ceiling, any ceiling, before I came to the Annex. But for the past couple of years, three or four mornings a week, at various times between 5:30 and 6:30 a.m., I lie on the small patch of bright green Astroturf or the hard rubber mats that make up the Annex's floor and I stare up, toward the roof. Sometimes it's the idle, thousand-yard stare of someone who has been awake for a mere fifteen minutes and is fighting to gain consciousness even as he tries to unlock his stiff and unresponsive muscles with the foam rollers, lacrosse balls, and rubber stretching bands laid out on the floor.

But more often it is the gaping-eyed, almost-panicked stare of someone who has just finished a workout that has taxed my brain, my spirit, my lungs, my guts, and every fiber of muscle in my body and has left me sprawled on my back on the floor, arms and legs spread-eagle, my chest heaving in a desperate, redlined fight for breath as sweat pours off every inch of skin.

That's the case this Tuesday morning. The 5:30 class, made up today as on most days of eight largely silent men ranging in ages from thirty-two to fifty-one and coached by a twenty-four-year-old former collegiate lacrosse player turned J. Crew stylist, has spent the last fifty-two minutes burning through a routine that starts with a warm-up that begins slowly with stretching and builds to a jump-roping crescendo as challenging as many workouts I'd done before I found CrossFit. (Or, as a T-shirt worn by one of my fellow travelers says, "Our Warm Up is Your Workout.") The warm-up is followed by an Olympic weightlifting session in which we do five sets of repetitions each of a lift called a back squat, which calls for us to put a bar loaded with as much as our body weight on our upper back while we drop under it into a squat before standing up. Then, and only then, does the real workout begin. Today, we are to do as many rounds as we can in fifteen minutes of the following three exercises: jumping from a dead stand still onto a 24-inch box ten times, swinging a 42-pound ball of steel with a handle called a kettle bell between our legs and over our heads ten times, and performing ten burpees, perhaps the single worse exercise in the CrossFit repertoire, a move that calls for us to throw ourselves prone onto the ground then leap back up into the air, clapping our hands over our heads.

I do CrossFit three or four times a week. And almost without fail, I find myself sprawled on the floor afterward. Some quick math shows that to be somewhere around two hundred opportunities to study the ceiling of the Annex in the past year, to learn its intricacies while life, in the form of precious oxygen, seeps back into me. I have noticed that as the year has progressed my sessions on the floor have gotten shorter, at least the ones at the end of the workout. That's a sign that my body is adapting to the rigors of the workout. I'm getting in shape. Which is the point. But I'm rarely happy with my performance. I can almost always find something to tweak, someone to beat.

In some ways, the warm-up is the worst part of the hour. Most mornings, not fifteen minutes before I start my routine on the floor, I am still in a perfectly warm bed. The alarm sends a staticky reminder to get up. I slump into shorts and a T-shirt, maybe a sweatshirt if it's cold, and drive the 3.3 miles from my house to the Annex. I do not drink coffee beforehand, for almost certainly I'd puke it back up mid-workout, which I'd figured out the hard way. For most of the year, I drive Shunpike Road in darkness, greeted by the inkling of dawn only in summer. My muscles stiff from sleep, middle age, and the last workout, the warm-up serves as a way to gradually work out the kinks, raise my body's internal temperature, and get my heart and lungs going. As such, I approach it very deliberately.

There's a digital clock at one end of the gym, one that dictates and defines everything that happens there. The fact that the clock is sold by a company called Again, Faster, speaks louder than anything what CrossFit is all about. Repeat it, and do it better this time. At 5:32, or 5:33, the coach will call out, "All right, guys, let's get started," and we'll slowly put away the foam rollers and bands we were using to coax life into our muscles. We'll gather at a small whiteboard near the turf and look at a list of exercises designed to get us moving, and ready to do the much harder work to come.

First comes twenty yards of what someone, somewhere, decided was the World's Greatest Stretch, or WGS. You toe the duct-taped mark at one end of the turf field, and lift one leg so you can hug that knee to your chest. Every muscle in that leg responds, sometimes groaning at the exertion, sometimes purring with the gentle call to life. You then shoot that leg forward into a long lunge, with the other leg splayed out behind you, and then twist gently at the waist to one side, then the other, loosening up your midsection and your hips. You take the elbow of the arm closest to your forward leg and try to touch it to the ground, down near that foot, and then reach the other hand to the sky, stretching every muscle in the body. Then you stand up, slowly, and repeat the process, all the way down to the other duct-taped mark, ten yards distant. You turn around, and you go back.

There you pick up a four-foot section of white, narrow-gauge PVC pipe slightly thicker than a broom handle to do some pass-throughs and some overhead squats. You hold the pipe up over your head, arms spread wide. Shrug your shoulders, then rotate the pipe behind you, keeping your hands toward the ends of the pipe, toward your lower back so that your shoulders and chest open up wide. Pause for a second, then bring the pipe back over head and in front of you, toward your waist. Repeat this ten or fifteen times until your upper body is nice and loose.

Then assume the overhead position again, but this time, with your feet planted shoulder width apart, squat down, weight on your heels, the pipe overhead and slightly behind your head so that someone standing next to you can see your ears jutting in front of your arms. Stay down in this squat so that your hips and shoulders loosen up. Don't be afraid to hang out down there. Remember, you're warming up, loosening up. Keep the weight on your heels so that you can easily wiggle your toes or slip a magazine under them. Then, weight still on your heels and your elbows locked overhead, stand up, nice and slowly. Repeat the whole thing ten times or so. Your hips will be opened up and loosened when you're done.

Go back to the duct tape and bend over and touch your toes. Slowly, slowly, slowly inch your fingertips forward, forward until you are flat out like a plank. Yes, your hamstrings will scream at first, but that pain will dissipate as your body weight shifts to your arms and shoulders, which will take up the screaming duties. Perform a push-up, then, with your weight on your hands, start slowly walking your feet toward your hands so that you feel your hamstrings stretching again. Walk them in until you get them as close to your hands as your hammies allow. Stand up, shake it out, and repeat until you reach the distant piece of duct tape, then turn around and do it again.

All this is done to the sound of only music. Nobody is awake enough yet to carry on a cogent conversation besides assorted grunts of assertion that the warm-up hurts. The music playing at this point is usually something upbeat but not over-the-top hard-core—that comes later when the workout begins in earnest. If there is a conversation, it almost invariably is about a game from the night before. There are a few other Red Sox fans here, and one of them, JP, stays up to watch each Sox game. I don't know when he sleeps. Anne tells me there's more talking at later WODs. The 6:30 class has the benefit of an extra hour of sleep, and daylight, to stir conversation, and the 8:45 a.m. class, made up almost entirely of women, is noted for its chatty warm-ups. But at 5:30, we're all grunts and groans.

We're not done. Head to the rubber mats, near the clock,

which coach has set to count down from one minute. Pick up a jump rope and, as soon as the clock starts, commence bouncing up and over it like a boxer. You can probably get in 150 or so reps before the clock counts down. Miracle of miracle, it's been set to immediately count down from ten seconds, just enough time for you to drop into the CrossFit sit-up position—flat on your back, soles of your feet butterflied near your crotch, arms stretched out on the floor behind you—so that you can snap out sit-ups for the next minute, bringing your hands from the floor behind you to the floor in front of your feet. The clock resets, and you move to the push-up position. Your body is a plank, and your nose and chest touch the ground before your arms shoot up and your elbows straighten. "All the way up, all the way down," coach murmurs. One minute of push-ups is way harder than a minute of sit-ups. You then head to the pull-up bar, and do as many pull-ups as you can in a minute. That's not many for me, but I can get in ten good ones as long as I jump up to the bar each time.

Congratulations. It's been fifteen minutes, and you're sweating mildly, your breath a little hurried but not uncomfortably so. You're warmed up. You're ready to start your WOD, or Workout of the Day.

But first, grab the PVC pipe again and form a circle. It's time to go over the weightlifting move at the heart of the strength portion of the WOD. We do this before every weightlifting session, which take place four days a week.

If there is one consistent and persistent complaint about CrossFit, it is that the complex Olympic weight moves that form the basis of the regimen's strength exercises are simply too difficult to master properly, are not coached properly, and that too many people are trying to push too much weight too soon and are at risk of getting seriously hurt. It's a tough impulse to control. At the Annex, the coaches try to do so by stressing the importance of proper form, and by constantly preaching the mantra "master the move and the weight will follow." It's easy to say but hard to enforce when your pupils are aggressive middle-aged men, most of them titans of Wall Street who didn't achieve their posts in life by listening to people.

Yet here we are, with the plastic PVC pipes laid across our shoulders, as coach talks us then walks us through the fundamentals of a proper back squat. Feet shoulder width apart. Stand up straight. Chest and shoulders upright, like a proud gorilla. Weight on the heels so you can wiggle your toes; head and chest and shoulders up; don't let the knees go ahead of your toes. Squat all the way down so that the crease formed by your hip and leg is below your knee. Then stand back up, all the way up, so that you can push your hips forward by squeezing your butt cheeks together. That's a proper back squat.

So we move over to the weight racks, and some of us buddy up with guys who are doing similar weights. I work with Joe and Leo; Steve Gephart works with Gerry on massive amounts of weight done with flawless form; the Twins, Martin and Edwin, work together; and some of the new guys work alone or in pairs. We use empty 45-pound bars laid across our backs to continue the warm-up, getting used to the movement performed with a little bit of weight. Someone turns up the music and puts it on a slightly more aggressive, or at least upbeat, channel, like the Foo Fighters or AC/DC channels on Pandora. There's more talking now as everyone comes alive and wakes up, and more ball-busting mixed in with the shouts of encouragement as the loads increase. Five reps at 135 pounds, another five at 155 pounds, the clanks of the bars as the lifters resettle them on the stanchions, the exhalations of guys pushing up, straining, against the loads as "There Goes My Hero" blares and someone puffs "Fuckfuckfuckfuck" like the little engine that could. Then it's on to three sets of three, adding a little bit of weight each time. Sometimes a guy will rack the load and smile dreamily as stars fill the fringes of his field of vision, as if he had just taken a very, very big hit off a spliff. Sometimes a guy will drop down and rise, slowly, like a foal standing up for the first time just seconds after being born, his legs shaking and the bar tipping crazily to one side. And sometimes, but not very often, a guy will go down with a load and not be able to get back up without the help of his friends rushing to his aid to help him finish the lift.

Depending on the weight move, the load, and the

weather, lifting can be a gross, sweaty mess of caked chalk and slippery bars and mats. And even though some guys were squatting well over their body weights today, nobody seems too messed up by the lifting, just energized and ready to move on to the last part of the hour: the WOD.

One of the founding precepts of CrossFit is that the workouts should be constantly varied. So you'll never do the same exercises, let alone the same routine, in a given week. That means that one day, the WOD could take the average athlete 20 minutes or so to complete, while another day it could take 7 minutes, and on a third, 45 minutes. That continuous variation, combined with always trying to go as fast and hard as you possibly can, is the thing that drives such quick and profound results. Yesterday the WOD took around 20 minutes, and the day before, 13.5 minutes.

Today, we are to do as many rounds as we can in fifteen minutes of box jumps, kettle bell swings, and burpees. Box jumps require you to stand still, feet hip width apart, and to vault onto a two-foot wooden box, landing squarely and as silently as possible on the top. You then hop back to the ground. That's one rep. To complete a kettle bell swing, you stand with the bell dangling between your legs. By thrusting your hips as licentiously as possible, the bell will swing up and over your head until its bottom faces the ceiling before dropping back down near your crotch. Burpees, named for physiologist Royal H. Burpee, who invented the movement in 1939 as part of a fitness test, are familiar to anyone who took a middle school gym class in the 1970s: stand up straight, drop to the ground so that your chest hits the deck and your legs are straight out behind you, stand back up as quickly as possible, and jump up in the air and clap your hands over your head. A Google search of "burpees suck" returns 125,000 results; "I hate burpees" returns 215,000. Surprisingly low, actually. They are a foundation move of CrossFit and the single exercise I hate most.

But here we go, the clock set to count down from fifteen minutes, and the eight of us prepared to do ten reps of the three exercises—the thirty reps making one round—as many times as possible in that time. For some of us, it's a race. Steve Gephart, Joe, Leo, and Dave will watch each other with guard-dog eyes and do everything they can to beat one another. Gerry, a former Ivy League champion shot putter, is, at six foot five and 220 pounds, the strongest of us but not the most fleet. The Twins are relatively new and will drown in their own sweat before they quit but are no match for the first four. I try to stay within myself, not watching the others or worrying about my place relative to everyone else, and yet I can't stand to lose, or to shake the feeling that if I am not in the lead, I am failing. I am never in the lead. Hence every morning, despite the visible and quantifiable improvement in my results over the years, at some point in the workout I will feel as if I am failing.

Tony, the coach today, turns up the music as he switches to a Metallica station at Gephart's request. He points the remote control timer at the clock and counts down. "In three, two, one, GO!" at which point we all begin bounding from the turf to the top of the boxes. Some land silently and stand up straight, hips fully extended, before stepping back down, one rep complete. Some bound as if they were jumping rope, the tips of their toes kissing the edge of the box before they hop down only to bounce up again, immediately. I am more deliberate, depending more on a vigorous arm swing and a "thumbs . . . UP!" mantra to propel myself squarely onto the box top before stepping down, trying to remember to alternate legs when I initiate the dismount.

The first ten are a breeze, as are the kettle bell swings. They look like an arm exercise, but the key to getting the weight squarely up and over your head is to squat down, weight dangling pendulously like a distended testicle, and to thrust your hips forward as if you were making extremely vigorous love, squeezing your butt cheeks when the weight reaches the top. (There is a lot of butt-clenching in CrossFit.) The arms and wrists control the weight, and the momentum.

Burpees are a different story. Such a seemingly mundane exercise takes up an awful lot of space in my head, and I approach them with dread. One of the truisms of CrossFit is that you should do the thing you hate most, because it's only in mastery that the hate will dissipate. I'd like to say I was fully in touch with my inner Shaolin priest, but I'd hate to lie. I throw myself on the ground, trying to not waste my arm and chest energy by lowering myself. I then push up, bring my knees up to my chest, stand up, do a slight hop, and clap my hands over my head. Positively awful. Ten times, and the first round is done.

By the time the second round starts, I'm warmed up nicely, feeling pretty good and noticing out the corner of my eye that Joe, Dave, and Leo are already on to kettle bell swings. I bound up and down, lactic acid starting to make its presence known in my calves and quads. Whenever I do box jumps, I stare warily at the rough edge of the box. It's a mark of honor among CrossFitters to have angry scabs on your shins, either from barking them against that edge when the jumping gets hard, or by scraping barbells against them during dead lifts. Chicks may dig scars, as the saying goes, but they hurt, so I take my time and reset to make sure I clear the landing.

By the time I move on to the kettle bells, my breath is coming in ragged bursts, so I put my hand on my knees and exhale hard three times before grabbing the bell and humping it for all it's worth—sharp exhalations get rid of the carbon dioxide rapidly building up in my system and help me gain my breath. Then I fall into the burpees, which are nothing but shittiness. I have yet to learn a mind trick that helps me endure these things, which cause my shoulders, deltoids, and abs to scream in fatigue.

Two rounds down, nine minutes to go.

At the box, I take a step up to start the first one. Technically, this is cheating. I am now performing a step-up, not a box jump, but I'd rather keep moving than stop to catch my breath. So much of CrossFit is a giant calculus problem in which you try to figure out the precise rate of movement or amount of weight so that you can perform as much work as quickly as possible. I might not even be aware of the fact that I'm performing the calculations, but I am, like a race car driver unwittingly solving complex equations as he figures out the fastest line through a turn. I resume the jumps on the third rep, and they are starting to get harder. I use a more aggressive arm swing now, spraying sweat from my arms as I swing them forward, painting the wall with a Pollock plume of briny drops of perspiraton. When I grab the kettle bell, the handle is slick with my sweat, so I pause to rub gymnastic chalk on my hands, as Leo has done before me. When I move from the swings to the burpees, my hands leave a telltale white paw print on the turf.

Each round gets a little slower than the last; each box jump requires a deeper lean and harder swing. The kettle bells don't seem harder, and I'm able to do them without pausing—"unbroken," in CrossFit parlance, a point of pride. The burpees become slower and more miserable, my jump microscopic, my clap barely audible, until Tony, whose exhortations have been lost on me all this time, says the words we all want to hear.

"Three, two, one, TIME!"

At which point I sprawl on the floor, five rounds complete, sweat searing my eyes, lactic acid burning my entire body, eyes sealed shut.

Slowly they open.

And there, on the ceiling, is a wire, copper jutting from its end. Going nowhere. A new detail on the tapestry of the ceiling. My chest heaves. My mind wanders. Most guys my age are still in bed at this time of day. Maybe they're snoring. Maybe they're pressing into their wife's back, hoping she'll wake up with the same thought he has. That's where I should be. But I'm here.

Slowly, we recover and walk to the whiteboard, where we write down our names and the number of rounds and reps we completed. Gephart, Joe, and Leo are way ahead of me. Gerry and I have tied. Only the Twins and a new guy are behind me. I didn't fail, but I didn't win.

That's what I'll remember for the rest of the day.

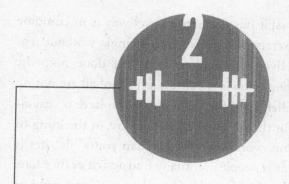

# How and Why It Works

The principles and the movements that form the basis of CrossFit certainly aren't new. As long as people have been interested in the benefits of physical fitness, we have had sit-ups, push-ups, weightlifting, and running among us. And as long as high school wrestlers have struggled to make weight, high-protein, zero-carb diets have been shown to work.

What CrossFit has done in a novel way is to combine the various exercise disciplines into a single workout regimen that delivers tremendous results if done properly. Arguments about who is the fittest athlete of all are boring beyond all belief, even for those of us who have occasionally engaged in them. What often gets lost in the kung fu movie-style "my workout is harder than yours" debates is the fact that most people eventually find activities they like, and they stick with them because they get some kind of pleasure from them, whether it's the camaraderie of a golf game, the endorphin buzz of a run, the admiring glances that can result from weightlifting, or the sheer pleasure of bombing down a hill on a bike. If you like it, or like how it feels, you're more likely to stick with it.

But at some point in nearly every exercise routine, boredom sets in, usually around the same time that improvement seems to plateau. Such was my case in 2005. As the editor of *Bicycling* magazine, I had a duty to ride as many bikes as much as I possibly could. Sometimes this required riding them in far-off and very pleasant locales, like Italy and France. Sometimes it meant riding bikes so expensive, so evolved, and so precise that I, a dedicated but aggressively untalented recreational cyclist, had no right planting my fat ass on them. Sometimes it meant transporting bikes for testing purposes, meaning that the sum worth of the bikes on the roof of my car was double the sticker price of the little Mazda. I rode about four thousand miles a year, in all kinds of weather.

I loved it, for all the same reasons I had loved playing hockey as a kid. I felt free, and even if other riders were faster than I was, I still felt fast. I loved it so much in fact that despite the fact that the magazine regularly wrote about the benefits of cross training and weightlifting, I seldom did either, preferring a ride in the cold rain or a boring indoor trainer session to an hour of planks and stretching. I was one of the few people in the world—messengers, pro racers, rickshaw drivers—who could say with a straight face, "I get paid to ride a bike," and I was going to take full advantage.

But right after Christmas that year, I was lying on the couch, watching some meaningless college football bowl game and enjoying a bottle of Tapestry when I tried to get up to answer the phone. I couldn't do the simple sit-up required to get off the couch. So I used my arms and pushed myself up. Later, in bed, I mentioned the physical lapse to Anne. "You should read about this crazy new workout that was in the paper last week," she said, adding that it sounded really tough but that the people who did it swore by its results.

So I read "Getting Fit, Even if It Kills You" in the *New York Times* the next morning, and was intrigued.

Over the years I had flirted with various forms of what the article described. In the late 1990s, I had worked out once a week with the actor-turned-trainer Terry Londeree, who combined weightlifting, plyometrics, and ballet movement into a workout so rigorous I was once unable to get off a plane after a New York to Phoenix flight, so stiff and sore had he left me. And about the time our son, Luke, was born, in 2000, I was a regular at a Monday night class in our hometown, called "Boot Camp" and run by a trainer named Ron who told us he had been to BUDS, the brutal weeks-long screening tryout for would-be Navy SEALs. Of course, Ron was also unable to tell the difference between a lie and the truth, as he demonstrated time and again with his wife and various female clients of this particular gym, but he sure knew how to put together an hour of calisthenics and dumbbell exercises that would leave most of us so depleted we were unable to take our car keys out of our pockets. And I was the organizer of a lunchtime workout for my coworkers, the Power Hour, designed to get them doing new movements, beside the usual running and cycling.

I knew this stuff, loved it even, but I had never stuck with it. Something new always seemed to come along, something that I wanted to try. Like CrossFit.

I was also familiar enough with exercise and my own disposition to know that I wasn't in any danger of driving myself to rhabdomyolosis, the condition in which people work out so hard they break down their muscles so fast they end up in the hospital. I like to work hard, to bring the hurt, but I know the difference between the hurt of "Wow, I'm working really hard but when I stop this will go away" and the hurt of "Holy shit, my muscles are breaking down and I need to go to the ER now." But the workouts, which the *Times* described as "a high-intensity mix [of] gymnastics, track and field skills and bodybuilding, resting very little between movements," seemed liked an ideal complement to my regime.

So I decided I would mix some CrossFit in with my regular rides, most of which were taking place on indoor trainers that time of year. I went to Crossfit.com, which listed the daily workouts in a jargon I didn't understand, but which was easy to navigate and had a stunning library of video clips in which insanely fit and beautiful people demonstrated the exercises. My thought was that I could watch the videos and do the workouts in the meager gym I was building in my garage, or in the gym at work. Many of the exercises were easy enough in principle: sit-ups, push-ups, pull-ups, squats, bench presses. But some of them were Olympic weight moves, the kind most of us see only for twenty minutes or so every four years when, in between gymnastics and swimming, the Olympic broadcasters deign to show some tiny Turkish guy or massive Russian in an embarrassingly small unitard screaming and throwing kilograms (kilograms! how much is that in pounds?) around in some cool but absurdly hard-looking maneuver. The folks demonstrating the moves on the CrossFit videos, most of which seemed to be shot in someone's garage and which were narrated by an unseen man with a cowboy voice like the stereotypical airplane pilot, made the lifts seem easy. Effortless, even.

I figured I'd play to my strength and start with an overhead squat, taking advantage of the leg strength cycling had given me. In our garage, I picked up an empty 45-pound Olympic bar and hoisted it over my head, arms spread wide, feet slightly more than shoulder width apart, chest and shoulders up, just like the video said, and tried to squat down. But I didn't move. I spread my feet wider and tried again. This time I was able to move my butt a tiny way down toward the floor, maybe an inch or two. But the bar started to slip. I simply didn't have the overhead strength to keep the bar up, the core stability to keep the whole of my midsection intact, nor the flexibility in my hips to allow my butt to drop. I let go of the bar and bailed out.

So I moved on to the dead lift, which various websites told me should be of a weight equal to my body weight. I warmed up with a plain bar, squatting down and keeping—I thought—my lower back flat, not rounded, and lifted with my legs, then my back, then shoulders, just like they did in the online videos. No problem. So I slowly added weight, until I actually was able to lift two hundred pounds or so, right around my body weight.

The next day, prone in bed with a back that would not move, I vowed to learn the proper ways to do the Olympic moves, perhaps this time from a coach, but to adapt the other CrossFit workouts, the ones that didn't require much technique, and use them to become a stronger cyclist.

Slowly, over time, my garage began to look less like a bike shop and more like a gym. I bought weight plates and another big bar, friends gave me kettle bells, Anne bought a jump rope, and we began. The Power Hour became a twice-weekly workout that was an amalgam of things I picked up off Crossfit.com and exercises I had learned from various trainers like Ron, and Terry Londeree. Friends and friends of friends, notified by word of mouth, joined us in the garage as we did the Power Hour in all sorts of weather; we rang in New Year's 2006 with a workout that added up to 2,006 reps of twenty different exercises. It was 16 degrees. In summer, we took it to the pool, where we would swim fifty yards at a pop and then do push-ups on the deck.

And I noticed an improvement in my cycling. I was able to stay hunched over the handlebars longer now, thanks to my newly strengthened back. I had a little more pop in my legs when I wanted to sprint, and my shoulders didn't ache from leaning on the bars. And yes, I could get off the couch without using my hands.

But we weren't doing the Olympic moves, which were in some manner or form on the site every day. And the Power Hour lasted just that, an hour, when most of the workouts on Crossfit.com seemed to average around fifteen minutes. I knew by now that whoever was putting the workouts together knew what he or she was doing, but I couldn't figure out why they thought you could get in shape—real shape—if you worked out for only twenty minutes. If there had been a CrossFit gym near me, I would have started going, to learn more about the right way to do all this. But there wasn't.

So I decided to attend a two-day CrossFit certification class, to learn the theory and practice behind the workout. Or, more to the point, I talked about doing it, but Anne actually signed me up and gave me a piece of paper on Christmas morning 2007, telling me I was going to Malvern, Pennsylvania, for a weekend in February to become a CrossFit-certified trainer.

The group of thirty or so people that gathered at Malvern Prep, a private boys school in suburban Philadelphia, early that cold Saturday morning was a mirror-accurate reflection of the types of people pictured on Crossfit.com at the time. Mostly thirty-year-old men, with a few women scattered in. Lots of tattoos and heads that were either shaved or sporting a neat number-two crew cut. T-shirts with skulls and crossbones and mantras about going hard or going home, socks pulled high up to the knees, baggy shorts. We went around and introduced ourselves to the group. There were a lot of engineers, some teachers, and a professional squash player and a professional racquetball player. There were a few trainers, too. At forty-four, I was one of the three oldest people there, and was absolutely mortified at having to do a workout, let alone demonstrate a lift, in front of any of these people, who almost all looked rabidly fit. But that wasn't really the point, I told myself. I was there to learn how to do this stuff right, and to finally learn some of the underlying theory behind it all. I told myself as the class started: This is about you, not them. It's not a competition. Get the benefit of it. Stay focused on yourself.

The class was taught by Tony Budding, straight from CrossFit headquarters in Santa Cruz, California. Budding looked like most of the guys sitting around me, but was far more physically imposing, even in a dark hoodie. He started by giving us a little bit of the history of CrossFit: Founded in 1995 by Greg Glassman, a former gymnast and trainer in Santa Cruz, as a counterintuitive way to train the county's sheriffs. At a time when everyone else in the "fitness industry"—a phrase Budding practically spat—was preaching the value and virtue of long bouts of "aerobic" exercise, "core" workouts, and calorie counting, Glassman was combining weightlifting and gymnastics moves with gym-class oldies like push-ups, squats, and sit-ups, forcing the body to use large muscle groups in concert, the way you would in real life. He urged people to go hard, all out, and that the workouts almost always be timed to take advantage of the competitiveness most people drawn to such a workout would naturally bring with them. In 2000, Glassman launched Crossfit.com, posting the workouts for free and widening the size of his flock as adherents looked up the workout of the day, posted each night at midnight Pacific time, then posted their performance stats in the comment sections after completing the WOD.

All of which had led us here, to Malvern. This was just one of more than ten certification classes ("certs" in CF parlance) taking place around the country this weekend, he told us. When we were done, we would understand a few truths, at least as CrossFit saw them: "You'll see that the fitness industry in this country is full of shit," Budding said. "Isolating a single muscle is bullshit. Biceps curls are bullshit." We would understand that it is better to train your weaknesses than it is to develop your strengths. We would understand that we were not training to become fitness specialists, more like jacks of all trade. And finally, Budding said, we would learn what CrossFit was trying to achieve: to prepare us all for whatever life asked of us.

I'm pretty sure he meant that in the physical sense. That if we were walking down the street and saw flames leaping from the windows of the top floor of a building, we'd be able to sprint up the fire escape, kick down the door, drag the obese man who had been overcome by the smoke to the door, throw him over our shoulders, and carry him to safety on the sidewalk. Or cradle one twin baby in each arm while descending to the cellar laundry room. Or do one power snatch every minute on the minute for forty-five minutes.

But I took it in a much more metaphysical way. That by working hard to eliminate my weaknesses, by pushing through a perceived barrier, by simply showing up and chipping away at the task, I could finish things and achieve my goals. And that if I could do it in a gym, I'd be able to do it at work, and at home, where three little kids demanded a constant stream of attention and work, and where Anne and I often felt overwhelmed by, well, everything. And maybe it would allow me to once and for all vanquish the voices in my head, telling me I wasn't good enough.

Budding explained a few things in what struck me as precise, if not stilted, language, some of which required some decoding on my part:

- "CrossFit is based on the principles of constantly varied functional movements done at high intensity." (Translation: We will always mix up the exercises and you will always go as hard as you can.)
- "Functional movements are natural, essential, elemental, safe, and efficient and effective." (Translation: They are not done on Nautilus machines; they allow you to live independently; they can't

27

be broken down further; you won't get hurt; and you'll get shit done.)

- "Movement categories include body weight control through space, external object manipulation, and monostructural activity." (Calisthenics and gymnastics; weightlifting; running, swimming, cycling.)
- "Fitness is an increased work capacity across broad time, mode, and age domains." (Translation: You can do more faster.)
- "Workouts fall into two categories: task workout, and time workout." (Translation: Do a certain workout and time yourself or do as much as you can in a given period of time.)
- "Strength workouts should be scary and hard. If you've done them right, you shouldn't be able to do a single rep more." (Translation: Lift until your muscles scream.)
- "Mechanics must be consistently good before they can be intense." (Translation: Learn how to do this shit right or you may get hurt trying to go hard.)
- "If you can't move the next day, you've done too much work." (No translation required.)

Budding delivered this information in a straightforward, no-nonsense way that made it very clear he had no doubt that he was right, and every other trainer in the world, the ones who would have you do twenty minutes on a treadmill, twenty minutes of crunches, and a few leg extensions while chatting to you about your upcoming vacation, was not only wrong, but was leading you down the path to morbid obesity, a depleted bank account, and an early death. And we took notes as if he were reading off the winning numbers in various state lotteries to be held in two weeks' time. (Had I paid such careful attention in college I wouldn't be writing for a living.) We were going to be fit, and healthy and happy. This guy had the answers.

I certainly was happy with the way they taught us the Olympic moves. We gathered in circles of ten or so in Malvern's gym, each of us equipped with a PVC pipe or broomstick. The instructors—one of whom had been an Olympic rower—would describe the movement to us, then demonstrate it very slowly, using the PVC as a stand-in for the weighted bar as he or she described it again. He'd then break the movement down into its constituent parts, citing mantras like "pop the pockets" or "weighted heels" or "dip and drive."

What became immediately apparent was that not only did I lack the strength to do some of these moves, but I also suffered from an appalling lack of flexibility. I had always prided myself on the flexibility in my lower body—I could bend over, straight-kneed, and easily put my fingertips and eventually my palms on the floor. But when it came time to put my two bended elbows straight in front of me, with the triceps parallel to the ground and my hands up by my face, I was useless.

Which led to another CrossFit truism: "Stretching is good. Do it." Something else to work on.

The moves actually got a little easier to perform when we put down the PVCs and broomsticks and used real weights; gravity, in some motions, was a big benefit. Only when deadlifting real weight—in which you go into a semi-squat with your hands on the bar in front of you and hips tucked under before standing and unfolding until you are upright and the bar and its load dangles mid-thigh—do you understand the true importance of good form. One bad lift, one misfire, and your back will let go in a second. "As a rule, your technique needs to be good, not great," Budding said. "B-plus, A-minus form is good enough. But you need to always be working toward A-plus form. It's the only way you'll get it, and the only way you'll get better."

I was just happy that I had enough information to do three basic lifts—the dead lift, the clean, and the push press—properly. Budding and other coaches went over the fundamentals of some of the more complicated exercises, like the glute-ham sit-up, which required a specialized piece of equipment that held the athlete's feet while she bent backward from the waist to touch the ground behind her before sitting back up. We also covered the wall ball shot, in which an athlete stands facing a wall with a medicine ball by his chest, squats down, then leaps up to throw the ball at a mark ten feet up the wall before catching it and dropping back into the squat. We learned about L sit-ups and the Holy Grail of CrossFit, the muscle-up.

A seemingly simple exercise, the muscle-up is a gymnastics move in which you reach up and grab a ring in each hand. You pull yourself up so your chin is above the rings, then work your hips and arms to drive yourself farther upward into a ring-dip position, with the upper half of your body above the rings, the rings down by your waist. Done properly, it is a display of mastery of everything CrossFit is trying to teach you: strength, coordination, agility, flexibility, endurance, speed. Get a muscle up and you have snatched the pebble from Master Po's hand; it is time to leave the Shaolin Temple. Until then, you work on it.

I was also happy that Budding talked a little bit about why going as hard as you can all the time leads to improved fitness. Most trainers and coaches would have you believe that athletes fall into one of two camps, aerobic or anaerobic. Or, distance guys and sprinters. And while it's true that people do have either predominantly fast-twitch muscles, the kind that make better sprinters, or slow-twitch, seen more in athletes with better endurance and less speed, very few adults train the sprinter muscles.

For one thing, going fast is hard, and it hurts. For another, according to Budding, the public has been brainwashed by the "fitness industry" and by doctors to believe that only a five-mile run or twenty-mile bike ride or half-hour continuous swim will produce health benefits, maintain healthy weight, or stimulate weight loss. Third, It had long been thought that an athlete was predestined by his biology to one kind of fitness or another.

But a body of research conducted by the Japanese physiologist Izumi Tabata has found that athletes who perform high-intensity interval workouts develop both their anaerobic and aerobic systems and burn fat, while those who train merely their aerobic systems develop only the aerobic system and can actually maintain or gain fat. So central is Tabata's research to CrossFit that Tabata has a WOD named after him, Tabata Something Else, in which athletes go as hard as they can at a particular exercise, say, squats, for twenty seconds, then rest for ten seconds for a total of four minutes, before performing the same routine with three more exercises. Done properly, it can be crippling, in a good way, as we learned when we did Tabata Something Else as one of the four WODs the instructors had us do over the course of the weekend. The last time something so brief had hurt so much was in eighth grade, when Ella Michaelson told me before school one day that she'd be my girlfriend but broke up with me at lunch.

Now, you can't go as hard as you can for four minutes over a period of twenty minutes, but the benefits still accrue. But form will suffer, and with bad form comes the possibility of injury. So with a few exceptions, most Cross-

Fit workouts don't last more than forty minutes, and most coaches will have an athlete stop if they haven't finished the work within that time. ("Murph" is a notable exception, see chapter 7.)

Over time, I would notice an additional benefit. When I came back from a long bike ride or run, or even a hike, I would be famished. The computer on my bike would tell me I had burned 1,500 calories, but if I wasn't careful, I could replace those calories and then some with a single sandwich and a handful of cookies. But the intensity of CrossFit not only placed a damper on my appetite; it brought, almost every time, an exercise-induced near-nausea that left me close to retching.

Budding spent a lot of time on nutrition, too. I wasn't approaching CrossFit as a means to weight loss, but it was becoming very clear that all this pulling up and running was going to be a hell of a lot easier at 180 pounds than at 200. And if I was going to sprout all these muscles, like the instructors, I might as well shed at least one of my layers of fat to show them off. As usual, Budding was very direct, starting his diet talk this way: "CrossFit has no commercial stake in nutrition. We don't benefit from trying to sell you anything." He added that CrossFit recommended the Zone Diet, Barry Sears's program, which dictates people eat a diet composed of 40 percent carbohydrate, 30 percent lean protein, and 30 percent "healthy" fat. "I guarantee obvious, fast, and dramatic results on the Zone," he said, before explaining how Zone Dieters weighed their food and apportioned it into blocks of each of the three nutrient groups. All the food was clean and unprocessed, and simple. But weighing food? I was neither a cheerleader nor Lance Armstrong, both of whom had been known to carry scales in their travels.

Rather, I decided to stick with the credo that had served me pretty well for many years: don't eat shitty food. What's shitty food? If it comes in a box, has a commercial, or is made in a plant, chances are it's shitty. (If it's advertised during the Super Bowl, it's really shitty.) If it just fell off a tree or was pulled from the sea, chances are it's not shitty.

At the end of the weekend, I sat in a corner and studied my notes. If I was reading this right, I would be able to spend less time working out, and possibly lose weight, all while getting muscles that had eluded me most of my life. I just needed to give it a try, and to stick with it. But in order to do that, I needed to find a box. My garage was great, but if this was going to work, I needed to find a proper CrossFit gym.

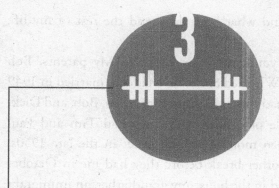

# That Fleeting Feeling

Two humid nights in August 1977, the month Elvis died, have defined my entire life. On the first night, on a weedy practice field in suburban Canton, Massachusetts, I discovered something about myself, in the process running away from a past that had identified me as someone I didn't want to be. On the second, on a football field in Norwood, Massachusetts, I announced who

I now was, and what I would spend the rest of my life trying to be.

I am the youngest of six children. My parents, Bob Madden and Winifred Shannon Madden, married in 1949 and by 1953 had three children: Maryellen, Bob, and Dick. After a couple of miscarriages, they had Tim and Paul within fourteen months of each other in the late 1950s, then took another break before they had me in October 1963. We lived in the house my grandfather, an immigrant from County Sligo, Ireland, built on Templeton Street in the Boston neighborhood of Dorchester, in St. Mark's Parish. My earliest memories are of three college-age siblings so much older than I that they seemed more like an aunt and uncles, and of the two brothers with whom I shared a room who were willing to throw batting practice to me for hours on end and to play basketball in the narrow driveway court wedged between our house and the Grahams' house, as long as the dribbling of the ball didn't disturb Jack Graham's sleep, because he was a farebooth attendant for the MBTA and worked odd hours.

There was a gang of kids my age in the neighborhood, and we played games incessantly. Not just sports like street hockey and Wiffle ball, but games like hide-and-seek, manhunt, Simon Says, and red rover. They all involved movement and physicality and play.

And I sucked at them, just like I sucked at baseball, basketball, swimming, tree climbing, and jumping the backyard fences that delineated our neighborhood. I was the fat kid. I would much rather stay inside and play with my Lincoln Logs, my Matchbox cars, or my Legos, patiently building cities with shoe boxes and cylindrical Quaker Oats containers on our living room floor, implausibly wearing grooves in my dad's LP copy of Stan Getz's *Jazz Samba* and then destroying the cities with an epic and purely imaginary windstorm delivered with a sweep of my arm.

My mother would urge me to go outside and play with the other kids in the neighborhood. When I resisted, she'd throw me out and tell me to not come home until dinner. So I'd go out—and play with my Lincoln Logs, Matchbox cars, and Legos in the dirt strip between the cool concrete of the driveway. I wouldn't say I was lonely. It was hard to live in a house with that many people and ever be alone, and I liked my brothers, who were genuinely good big brothers to me. But they were just that much older than me, tweens when I was in grade school, and not that interested in always palling around with the baby. And the other kids? They were running around, chasing each other, and playing games and sports, and I sucked at them. The way my eight-year-old mind saw it, why would I do something I sucked at? The cities I built with Lincoln Logs and Legos were huge, sprawling, complex affairs, a masterpiece of the child planner's art. When I played with my cities, there was nobody to keep up with, nobody to measure myself against, nobody to tell me I was fat and slow. And I liked it that way.

But my mother didn't. And unknown to me, she and my dad were fighting about me.

My mother, tired of having to buy my clothes in the Husky Boy section of Jordan Marsh, wanted to sign me up for youth hockey. My father didn't want to. He didn't want the expense. He didn't want the pain in the ass of having to drive me to the rink every Saturday. And he didn't want me to get hurt. My father was an only child, and as my mother told me when I was in high school and all this came to light, a real "momma's boy," who ran track but wasn't allowed to play football or hockey. He was an enthusiastic spectator, but he never got in the game, something that I now realize carried over to every aspect of his life. He was content to watch other people live.

My mother wasn't. She had been an open-water swimmer as a teenager, an Irish-American Gertrude Ederle, pulling on an itchy black wool bathing suit, coating her skin with a layer of lanolin, and wading into the frigid water of Boston Harbor to swim a couple of miles. Her sisters, happy to sit on the beach and smoke cigarettes, made fun of her big shoulders. She didn't care. Later, I remember her pulling on a black leotard and riding the Red Line to Cambridge to do a ballet class called the Joy of Movement taught by a Russian émigré named Mrs. Spora. She reveled in the physical at a time when women, especially in our working-class Irish neighborhood, were supposed to stay home and be den mothers to Cub Scouts. Had Jane Fonda released her exercise videos ten years before she did, I'm sure Ma would have worn leg warmers. And I'm sure my father would have mocked her. And I'm sure she would have worn them anyway.

In short, Ma was a badass and Dad wasn't. And she was damned if she was going to let her overly cautious husband blow this, her last chance, to have a kid who really got in the game. Not that my siblings didn't play sports, but my dad steadfastly refused to let my brothers play football or hockey or to swim, in short, to do anything that would require his participation, either financial or temporal, despite the fact that he was burstingly proud that a high school teacher had once remarked that Bob had a great pair of hands, after watching him play an intramural game.

That all changed one day when I was in third grade and Ma announced that she had signed me up for hockey. It was a problem. I couldn't skate, and we had no equipment. "Doesn't matter," she said. "You have to start somewhere."

Somewhere turned out to be on my ass on the ice at a rink in Squantum, Massachusetts, that was housed in an old airplane hangar. I would struggle to do a lap, using my stick as a tripod as the other guys zoomed around me. That the sessions were at noon on Saturday meant we could stop by McDonald's for lunch afterward, and was a big inducement, but I also just plain enjoyed it. Little by little, week by week, I got better, and had a huge breakthrough when my brother Bob and his fiancée, Beth, took me to a frozen golf course pond and showed me ice-skating was more about gliding on the blades than walking.

I played in the Neponset Youth Hockey League's house league for the next five years. The house league was the province of kids who just wanted to play but weren't good enough to compete. The travel teams, A and B, were reserved for the studs, whose flashy uniforms and new skates we hand-me-downers eyed with envy. The kids on the travel teams seemed to even have better hair than us scrubs in the house league. We skated once a week, usually Sunday mornings at six in a searingly cold open-air rink in Dorchester. As soon as I would come off my shift, I wanted to go back on. It was all explosive movement and speed, a speed I lacked when I tried to run. Games were an hour. I loved them, and lived for them.

Because when I skated, really and truly skated the way Bob and Beth had taught me to on that pond, all of a sudden I wasn't slow, and being fat didn't matter. Something alchemic happened when the blades of my skates played over the ice. Whatever combination of musculature, bone structure, and physics that made me slow and awkward on grass or pavement disappeared when I was on ice. In fact, I was one of the fastest in the house league. I scored goals. I blocked shots. And the weight that drove me to the Husky Boy shop was now ballast I could combine with my speed to pin kids against the boards. Nobody was inviting me to play for the travel team, but it almost didn't matter. I was, compared to the other kids in the house league anyway, fast.

But on Templeton Street, nobody else played ice hockey, so nobody could see the new me. Especially the Hatfield brothers, Billy and Bobby, my new friends from up the street but also, in the way of boyhood friendships, my rivals. The Hatfields were almost feral in their athleticism. They could climb higher than anybody else in the huge tree in Eddie Beal's backyard, swinging from limb to limb to the ground like urban Tarzans. Their snowballs, thrown with deadly accuracy and adult velocity, hurt more than anybody else's. They could get over fences simply by placing a hand on the tops and vaulting over. They were wild and funny and fun to be around, and I did everything I could to get them to play cards or Monopoly or Matchbox cars, because when we did that, I wasn't slow and awkward and left standing at the base of the tree, staring up at them in the far branches. I could win at Monopoly.

The Hatfields' parents were divorced. Bobby and Billy lived with their mom and two sisters, and their dad was never around. But their uncle Paul, a single guy in his twenties, would come every weekend and take them to the suburbs, pitching batting practice or throwing long bombs to them on the carefully groomed fields of Milton Academy, a prep school about five miles from Templeton Street that may as well have been on the other side of the world. Sometimes I got to go with them, and the three of them would reinforce—with every pitch blown by me, or every pass I couldn't haul in—just how bad I was at sports.

Until it got cold. Then the activity switched to pond hockey, and our roles reversed. The Hatfields were slow and uncoordinated and weak-ankled on skates, while I poked the puck between their legs only to retrieve it behind them after I had skated casually around them to head up the ice and score. I could skate backward on defense and break up their passes, then rush the length of the small pond to lay the puck between the two shoes we had set up as a goal. And when I did, I saw the look on their faces—frustration, anger, dismay, and maybe some despair—that I recognized from my own face almost every afternoon on Templeton Street. I was careful to never rub in the fact that I was better at ice hockey than they were. I didn't have to. They knew. And so did I.

Now I knew what it felt like to be good at something. To win. I had never known it before, and I wanted to feel it all the time, in everything I did.

Just after I completed seventh grade, we moved. My parents, especially Ma, despaired as our neighborhood decayed around us. Part a victim of 1970s white flight, part a victim of the court-ordered school desegregation plan that turned Boston's streets into rock- and broken-glass strewn battlefields, our once staunchly blue-collar Irish neighborhood was being taken over by what my siblings called another colored group: white trash. I had never heard the phrase before, but took it to mean the Hells Angels who got drunk on hot summer nights and waved their pistols from the roofs of the three-deckers across the street from us.

My parents sold the house for what I'm sure was a loss and bought another one on a busy street in Canton, a suburb about ten miles from Dorchester. We moved a couple of days after *Star Wars* debuted. There were no kids my age in the new neighborhood; there wasn't much of a neighborhood at all. I was bored. This time, I was lonely. I was angry at my parents for making me move, for leaving a school I loved. For leaving kids whose every physical action may have made me feel inferior, but who were still the only kids my own age I had ever known.

But it turned out to be a blessing. With nobody to hang with—and nobody to measure myself against or to lose to—I started running. The jogging boom was in full swing, so I borrowed a pair of my brother's old sneakers and went to the track (a seemingly suburban invention because I had never seen a 440-yard oval) at Blue Hills Regional Technical School, just up the street from our new house. Sometimes I ran a mile. Sometimes I would run the length of the straightaway a couple of times. Sometimes I'd just walk. But I moved. In the absurd heat of late mornings in July and the humidity of August, almost every day for two months. There was no training, no goal. I was looking for something to do, and this suited me. I had found something that suited me. Alone, there was nobody to lose to. I didn't feel slow, or fast. I just felt the pleasure of movement, and the weird pleasure in the pain of going hard, a pain/pleasure ratio I would spend the rest of my life trying to understand, but always enjoy, as I did on those hot solo days on the track. Access to this maroon oval opened up something in me that was as valuable, and as elemental to me, as learning how to read.

I made my poor parents' lives miserable as I alternately pined for "home," as I thought of Dorchester, and pouted silently behind the closed door of my new room. One night I saw an ad in the *Canton Journal* for Canton Youth Football tryouts. I wasn't interested in playing football—the thought of being hit, repeatedly and on purpose, by another kid was actually terrifying. But I figured it would be a good way to meet some other boys before school started so that I didn't walk into the William H. Galvin Middle School on day one of eighth grade without some sort of wingman. I declared my intention to play football.

It was the first time I ever saw my parents fight. I had heard them fight before, from behind the closed door of their bedroom, where they conducted all of their business, but this was out in the open, around a new kitchen table. It was both fascinating and horrible to see my parents fight, and to know that I was the spark that had ignited the tinder that had gathered in the stress of the move from Dorchester. My mother was adamant that they should let me sign up. My father was equally set that I should not.

44

In a futile effort to convince my mother, he played all his cards at once: time crunch caused by a longer commute into the city; expense; travel to games on weekends, which was his only time to relax; my health and safety. It was ugly. But my father, who could bend his sons to his will with a single look over the top of a newspaper or a reach for his belt buckle, caved to Ma's cold stare. I was playing.

One Friday night, she dropped me off behind a school on Neponset Street. Now, in the modern age of parenting, when every parent stays for every practice and goes to every game, I have to wonder if it was hard for her to let me go, alone, into a group of kids and coaches she and I had never met, thinking it would be good for me. Or if she thought, That little shit has been a pain all summer. Have fun.

Whatever she thought, by the time she came to pick me up, I was a different person.

What I had learned in the previous ninety minutes changed everything. I was the fastest kid on the field. Not just fast, but big, too. Big in a good way. Not fat, but tall and strong. The tryout had consisted almost entirely of running, calisthenics, and catching passes. We ran sprints, and then we ran some more, and each time we ran I finished a little farther ahead of the kids who came in second and third. I had speed and endurance. Each time I ran, the coach, a short lawn maintenance guy named Eddie, would look at his stopwatch and ask me, "What's your name again?" or "Where did you say you were from?" The other boys, none of whom I knew, all of a sudden paid attention to me. The new kid in town was fast. I still don't know if the kids in Dorchester were a superior race of athletes bred to toughness by having to walk everywhere, and the suburban kids were weak and slow because their moms drove them everywhere, or if, more likely, the two months of working myself had finally developed in me a leg strength I was never going to get playing with Legos.

But that Friday night, I became an athlete. I was no longer fat. I wasn't slow. I wasn't uncoordinated. All of that had vanished in the first forty-yard dash, when I sped up the field, looked left and right and saw myself all alone. No Hatfields. No Husky Boy clothes. I had left that all behind on the track at Blue Hills Regional during those hot, solitary summer days.

Two weeks later, surrounded by new friends who had spent the last two weeks calling me and inviting me to their houses and to swim in their backyard pools, I found myself in the backfield during a scrimmage against the Norwood, Massachusetts, eighth-grade team. It was early evening, and the setting sun cast long shadows across the grass, making us all seem like the giants some of us were in our heads. I had no idea what I was doing beyond the fact that I was to take the handoff from quarterback John Homer and charge through a hole somewhere to the right of the center, near the tackle, Scott Sullivan.

John called the signals, the center snapped the ball, and suddenly it was in my hands. I ran toward Scott but there was no hole. So I ran to the outside. And ran, and ran. I was petrified someone was going to catch me, and that fear fueled my legs better than double espressos. Touchdown. The first time I carried the ball. The first play of the game. The first snap of the first game I had ever played.

I don't remember what happened on the set of defensive downs we ran next. I was too stoked by having been pummeled on the back by my friends and thinking, This is what it feels like to win. I had never felt it before, not to this degree. We were winning because I was fast. And I was fast because I had worked hard all summer.

On the next set of downs, Eddie called in the same play I had scored on. Only this time they were waiting for me and I had my head taken off. "Get down!" Eddie yelled. So the next time I got the ball, I stayed lower and got outside. First down.

Then Eddie called a play that had me going up the middle to the left. I was more tired than I had ever been in my life, but I knew it was coming to me and I wanted to keep the feeling alive. I got the ball, bounced off someone, headed left, and ran downfield.

Norwood chased me. The Hatfields were chasing me. My teammates, my new friends were chasing me. But none of them caught me. They couldn't. I was fast now. I was an athlete. I was winning. And if I was winning, I must be doing something right. Touchdown.

Later that hot night, I stood in the shower of that new-to-us house on Randolph Street, letting the water rinse away mud and grass stains and marveling at the bruises and welts on my body. I was too tired to lift my arms to wash my hair. I had never felt such fatigue, but nor had I felt such a happy feeling of knowing I had given everything I had to give, and of seeing—feeling—such a rich reward for the effort. It wasn't just the winning; it was knowing that I had tried my hardest and that what was inside was good.

So I pursued it with a fury. In high school, I continued with team sports: Football, more hockey, then track and soccer. I started bike racing in high school. And each and every time I started a new sport, I pushed the wedge between my parents a little deeper. When I announced I wanted to do a fifty-kilometer bike ride in Salem one Sunday in June 1980, my father flipped out. "Twenty bucks to do a bike ride? You could just ride from here for free!" he yelled. He had two speeds when it came to this stuff: redlined and stop. He was redlining now. The thought of spending money on something like exercise was enough to explode his Depression-era mind. I didn't blame him, not really. My father had known true hunger as a kid during the 1930s. But times had changed. Surely he could give me twenty dollars to do something healthy. It's not like I was going to blow it on weed and beer.

My mother stood behind him, silently waving a twenty-dollar bill, letting me know it was okay, she had me covered.

"And we'll have to get up in the middle of the night to drive you," he said.

Ma pantomimed driving a car. She'd take care of it.

"What makes you think you can ride fifty kilometers, anyway?" he finally spat.

"What makes you think he can't?" Ma suddenly snapped, outrage in her voice, as if the answer had been primed on her tongue since 1955, left unused during previous fights and previous sons on this very topic.

"What makes you think he can't?" she said again. There it was. The difference between the two people who had, together, defined me. She wanted an answer and he didn't have one. One of the core differences between my parents was being played out over me, in the kitchen. For the first time, I saw my parents not as a unit whose job it was to raise me, but as two individuals, with separate personalities, goals, ambitions, and styles. When I got older, I would wonder what the hell had ever brought these two very different people together. But for now, I simply marveled at the thought that they would fight over this, and in front of me, a kid.

They didn't speak for a couple of days. But all three of us drove to the race. I felt free and independent pedaling my Schwinn Varsity around Salem Green. The Olympic speed skater Eric Heiden, who had retired from that sport to race bikes, was there, and so was I. I was in the game.

It went on like this for years. Dad never accepted why I wanted to do this stuff, but as I did more of it, I grew bolder. When he grumbled about driving me two hours to the state championship track meet, I told him it could be worse—he could be driving to bail me out of jail. Here I was, an honor student going to the state championship, and all he could do was complain. "I'm so proud of you," Ma said, rubbing my knee. Whether it was for standing up to him or making the meet in the first place, I still don't know for sure. I imagine it was both.

Years later, as an adult, free to make my own decisions and pay my own way, I stopped to see my by-then elderly parents when I was en route to a climbing trip in Nepal. During a pre-departure dinner, Dad listed all the reasons why I shouldn't be going to Nepal: There were communists there. Why did I want to sleep on the ground for a month? He had slept on the ground for almost two years during World War II and it was no fun. Nepal had only one phone for every two hundred people. I ate my pie and told him I didn't know anybody there anyway and so had no need for a phone. Mom laughed. He scowled, and asked me how much my fancy new North Face jacket cost. I lied. "Send lots of postcards, okay?" Ma said, hugging me at the airport. "Have fun. And please come back."

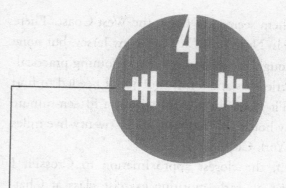

# Finding a Box

I f I learned anything at the Malvern certification weekend, it was that I needed more coaching, especially in the Olympic moves, the more complicated kipping style of pull-up that is a staple of CrossFit worlds and which would become my white whale, and of course the muscle up. I needed to find a box. Crossfit.com had a list of affiliate gyms where I could get the specialized coaching I needed, but most of them seemed to be on the West Coast. There were a couple in New York City and New Jersey, but none were close enough to my home to make joining practical. With three little kids and a full-time job, I needed to find a box (CrossFit-speak for a gym) within a fifteen-minute drive from my house in Chatham, about twenty-five miles west of New York City.

Until then, the closest approximation to CrossFit I could find was an early morning exercise class at Chatham's Annex Sports Performance Center. The Annex wasn't a gym in the traditional sense; you couldn't just walk in there and get on a StairMaster and go at it for thirty minutes. In fact, there were no StairMasters. Rather, the Annex was a serious training place for serious athletes run by a serious guy named Mickey Brueckner. A former major-league pitching prospect, Mickey is huge: six foot four and at least 250 pounds. If haberdashers should look fresh from the pages of *Esquire* and music store owners be able to pick up a guitar and play the beginning of "Stairway to Heaven," then gym owners should be as physically imposing as Mickey, who came equipped with muscular arms and legs and a barrel chest and back. He was fastidious to a fault, with never a hair out of place; any dumbbell left not racked in the proper ascending order of weight would cause him disgust, and, I suspect, some anxiety. He wasn't bulbous and cartoonish like a body builder; he was built to work. He looked as if he could do everything in the gym, and everything in the CrossFit playbook, even if the Annex weren't an official CrossFit affiliate.

Mickey could do everything except talk at 5:30 in the morning. Get him later in the day and he'd crush you with a handshake, call you his buddy, and warmly talk your ear off. But at this time of day, the best he could do was stand, arms crossed, and stare at us while we struggled to get our legs and hips to work in concert so early in the morning, mustering, at the best of a times, a brusque "Get that butt down there now."

Brueckner had found a sweet spot in the suburban economy, training high school kids whose parents had dreams of college scholarships for their budding lacrosse and baseball stars, or even bigger payouts in the pros, and the money to try to make those dreams reality. (He also trained a few professional athletes; their framed, autographed jerseys adorned the walls.) When school let out, the Annex was a hive of activity as kids arrived to lift, stretch, and bound their way to scholarships under the cold, analytical eyes of Mickey and his staff. A bulletin board bore testament to his work. Covered with newspaper clippings describing the achievements of his kids—championships, all-star teams, college scholarships—it was the first thing a prospective client and her parents saw when they came in the door of the Annex.

But at 5:30 a.m., it was the province of a few middle-aged men looking for nothing more than a way to beat back time and to stay in shape. We had all, in some way, heard about CrossFit and were looking for a way to get the benefit. We knew next to nothing about training, especially lifting, which was one of Mickey's specialties.

I didn't know it at the time, but the guys who showed up at the Annex for those workouts would form the core group of the 5:30 a.m. class, a core that endures to this day. Most of them had known each other for years. They were all successful, very fit, and hypercompetitive. Leo, a commercial real estate broker enshrined in the Lacrosse Hall of Fame and seemingly as fit in his late forties as he had been in his early twenties. Joe, my cycling buddy, who made up in power what he lacked in form or finesse and who had introduced me to this group. Jerry, a Master of the Universe who was once the Ivy League shot-put champion. Dave, a rabidly fit trash-talking CEO who thought nothing of getting off a red-eye flight and coming straight to the Annex for a workout. Steve Gephart, a former marine built like a fire hydrant, and who could throw around massive amounts of weight and preferred to do it to a deafening sound track of speed metal played at full blast.

When I first met these guys, I immediately had that familiar, sinking feeling that I was hanging around with the Hatfields again.

Mickey started us out with very basic exercises, the things Tony Budding had called "any-asshole" moves because any asshole off the street could do them. While the asshole part was not entirely true, they were the exercises in the CrossFit playbook that required the least amount of skill and coordination. These were familiar body-weight exercises like sit-ups, push-ups, air squats (an unweighted exercise in which you lower your butt to a medicine ball placed just behind you), and walking lunges. Working them into combinations, done at flank speed, could mess you up, and doing them properly, so that you got the full benefit and didn't risk injuring yourself, was way harder than it looked.

Take the walking lunge. Pretty straightforward: You shoot your right leg out in front of you, flexing the knee so that you drop your hips, descending until your left knee just kisses the ground. Be careful to keep your forward knee above the foot; if it goes too far in front, you could hurt the inner workings of the knee. Keep your upper body upright, and your hands off your legs—no leaning. Bring the left foot forward so you're standing straight up. Now shoot the left foot forward and repeat it. Sometimes you do this for 10 yards, sometimes for 50. Sometimes you do it while holding a 45-pound plate straight up over your head.

Devilish spins could be put on sit-ups and push-ups, too. Handstand push-ups are just that: you put your hands on the ground in front of a wall, flip yourself up so that your body is flush against the wall and you're in a handstand, then do push-ups while your butt and back slide against the wall. Or push-ups with your hands on gymnastic rings, your feet up on a box, maybe with some chains around your waist, just for a challenge. I could do them all, but not always as fast as the other guys could.

Any asshole? Any strong asshole, maybe.

Still, I found the skilled and semiskilled moves more intriguing, and some of them really hard to master. Like jumping rope, a foundation of many CrossFit WODs. I could jump rope all day long, as long as I wasn't trying to do anything fancy. Just bouncing along on my toes, hands down, lightly swinging the rope, no problem. But Joe could skip rope as well as any boxer, doing all sorts of tricks like holding the rope handles with a baseball bat grip and swinging it side to side. When I asked him where he learned to do it, he just shrugged. "I wrestled in high school," he said.

Joe was also the first one to master double unders. A CrossFit WOD never asks its athletes to jump rope. Rather, it asks them to perform a double under, which means that for every time you jump in the air, the rope passes under your feet twice. Sounds simple, but for some reason, I was confounded by it. While Joe could make the rope—really just a thin bit of plastic-covered wire with long handles— hum with the distinctive buzz of a double-under master as he pumped out 10, 20, 30 in a row, the rest of us would get one or two before slashing ourselves with the rope. While Joe's rope buzzed in taut circles, the other main sound in the room was the rest of us yelling variations, some of them operatic, of the F-word.

The trick to a double under is to bounce a little bit higher than you would when doing a standard rope jump, and to move your hands as fast as possible. Bending the knees as you jumped, into a tuck squat, didn't work. So you kept your legs pretty straight and you had to jump higher to clear two rotations of the rope. It was all about bounding high off your toes and moving your hands fast.

It took practice. Within a couple of weeks, I was able to string together 2, then 3, then 5 or 6, consecutive double unders. Rather than letting us scale—CrossFit-speak for reducing the workload by decreasing weight, bending the rules, or using some sort of mechanical aid to help an athlete perform an exercise—by performing, say, three regular jump-rope reps for every double under, Mickey insisted that we count attempts as reps. "If we stayed here until you guys got in all the reps," he said one morning, "nobody would get to work today. Just count your attempts."

That sort of practice is fundamental to the art of chipping away, a habit I learned early on, and one that helped me develop, if not perfect, the skills we were after. Rather than looking at a workout and thinking, My God, this is impossible, we're supposed to do one hundred burpee box jumps, I'd break it down into smaller, more manageable chunks: groups of ten reps with a three-breath rest in between, for example. Chipping away is so fundamental to CrossFit that "chippers" are their own category of WODs, usually composed of 25 or 50 reps of as many as 20 different exercises. You just chip away at a WOD like Filthy 50 (50 reps of 10 exercises) until you're done.

Some exercises and movements, however, seemed to be immune to the chipping away, at least for me.

I'd always had a problem with pull-ups, going all the way back to junior high. Pull-ups differ from chin-ups in that the hands face away from the body, pretty much eliminating the biceps as a source of power in the move. Like most people, I could always do more chin-ups than pull-ups, but try as I might, I simply lacked either the coordination, the upper body strength, or the willpower to perform more than a few pull-ups in a row before having to let go of the bar and drop to the ground. I had read once in *Outside* magazine that the great American alpinist Alex Lowe would do four hundred or more pull-ups a day, but his nickname was the Mutant, so that put him out of my league. And when I found an article online that doubted the value of pull-ups as a measure of true physical fitness—the physiologist argued that you could either do them or you couldn't, depending on your God-given morphology—I figured that was all the license I needed and dropped them altogether from my fitness routines.

Whatever your morphology, though, if you want to do CrossFit you are going to do pull-ups. They are an elemental move, and come in a couple of varieties. There are strict pull-ups, which require you to hang from the bar and pull yourself up until your chin is above the bar, then to lower yourself until you hang from fully extended arms and pause before you pull yourself up again. You may not rock your hips or legs at all while performing a strict pull-up. (If there is anything in the world to make you want to lose twenty pounds, short of a TV appearance in a swimsuit, it's the experience of hanging from a pull-up bar and trying to get just one more rep. You will feel every Dorito and pint of Sam Adams you ever drank while you try to get your head up over the bar.)

There are chest-to-bar pull-ups, in which you bring your chest, rather than your chin, to the bar. There are jumping pull-ups, in which you stand on the ground, jump up to grab the bar, and pull yourself up before letting go and dropping to the ground before repeating. There are burpee pull-ups, in which you perform a burpee under the bar and rather than simply jumping up to clap your hands above your head, you jump up and grab the bar to finish with a pull-up.

And there are kipping pull-ups. Reminiscent of a routine on a gymnastics high bar, kipping pull-ups are part regular pull-up, part hip drive, and part kick, all in the name of getting the chin above the bar while maintaining enough momentum to do the next one and the next one and the next one. While strictly speaking it isn't really a pull-up, the kip requires a high degree of strength and coordination. It also requires a flexibility and power in the hips that I didn't have. Some people can watch an instructor rip out a few kips then step right up and do them. Every one of the core group of the 5:30 class could kip like an Olympic gymnast.

Not me.

When I first tried to kip, under Mickey's direction, I hung from a bar and rocked my hips.

"Not your knees," Mickey said. "Start from the hips."

"I am."

"No, you're not."

I'd never felt like more of a motor moron than I did flailing on that bar. He had me jump down, lie on the floor, and initiate a hip thrust. This was at 5:45 a.m., with other grown men watching. I looked more like I was gatoring at a fraternity brother's wedding than seriously training. I wanted to get up. Mickey wouldn't let me until I had flopped in a way that he—and only he—seemed to think was close to a kip.

It's a central tenet of CrossFit that you are to leave your ego at the door when you enter a box. There is simply too much to master for any one person to think he can do everything. It's the sort of thing I had hoped I would have accepted, especially after grappling with my own subparness for a lifetime. But even though I knew I needed coaching—had, in fact, sought it out and was paying for it—I still felt like I had been called in front of the class to solve a particularly easy math problem on the chalkboard, one that everyone else had got on the first try and I alone couldn't do.

Back on the bar, Mickey's instructions weren't taking. "Push back from the bar!" Leo yelled.

"Get horizontal!" yelled Dave.

I jumped down and grabbed a giant white rubber band, knotted it over the bar, and put my foot through. Like a slingshot, it rocketed me up until my chin was over the bar.

"That's not a kip," Mickey said.

"You're cheating," said Leo.

Dave said nothing.

I had work to do. Every time I went to the Annex, regardless of the workout, I would try to end my session with ten pull-ups. I installed a Stud Bar in my garage so I could practice at home, bought my own rubber bands, and did everything I could to chip away. I worked on climbing the ten-foot ropes that dangled from the Annex's ten-foot ceiling, mastering the wrapping of the rope around my right leg and foot so I could stand on it with my left foot, inchworming my way to the ceiling, developing upper body strength I prayed would help my pull-ups. I got marginally better.

If only I were lighter, I thought. They'd come to me. If only I weren't the fat kid.

I faced the same issue with the muscle-up. I knew from my time at the cert that a strict muscle-up was out of the question. I lacked the upper body strength and hip drive to simply stand on the ground, pull myself up, and drive through into a ring dip. But if I jumped, vaulting up as forcefully as I could with a ring in each hand, I was able to at least pull myself up so my hands were at chest level.

Mickey agreed it was a good start, and decided we would break down the muscle-up into its component parts—starting with the pull-ups. Awesome. Muscle-ups are made more difficult by the fact that they're done on rings dangling from straps rather than a fixed bar. The fact that the rings move independently means that you can apply more force to your stronger, more dominant side. But it also means that the ring on your weaker side can squirt away from you, leaving you hanging in midair from one ring.

After watching a few of these, Mickey had another idea: he moved the rings to waist height and stretched the thick rubber band, the kind I had used for pull-ups, between the two.

"Grip it between your fingers, then press down on it with the heel of your hand against the ring," he said, showing me. I did as he said. The band, now stretched taut between the two rings, made a playground swing of the apparatus.

"Now hop up and sit on the band," he said. I did. The band sagged a bit under the load of my ass.

"Now lean back so you're lying flat." I did that, too.

"Okay, I want you to snap your hips really fast so that you're sitting up, and as you do, drive through the straps and down on the rings so you come into a dip position," he instructed.

It was the first time that a relatively difficult CrossFit move—even a scaled one—came to me right off the bat. I laughed with glee, the way I'd seen some people do when they get their first double under or rope climb. And I immediately wanted to do it again. And again. And again. Like I was twelve years old and playing hockey. All I wanted to do was move on to the real rings, to try a real muscle-up. A real muscle-up was the equivalent of making the travel team.

But real muscle-ups were as hard for me to get as a kip, and I soon figured out it was because of a lack of coordination—"putting it all together," as Mickey said. I had all the component parts, more or less: the pull-up, the drive, the dip. It was just a matter of getting them to work together. Something else to practice, another bogeyman to drive away. Another thing to watch the other guys do. Another thing to chip away at.

The Olympic weight moves proved to be less problematic, and of all the things I learned in CrossFit, the Oly lifts were the most satisfying, the most fun, and the most gratifying. Because when done properly, nothing makes the entire body feel like a glowing torch quite like a hanging snatch.

Why? Because it takes your entire body to perform the lifts. You might get bigger by isolating a certain muscle with an exercise like a biceps curl, but when in real life do you ever make the same motion as a biceps curl, at least outside of a pub? You don't.

The Olympic moves, on the other hand, require a progressive involvement of all the body's major muscle groups. You may be particularly sore in your shoulders and lats after a hard round of cleans, but you can be sure that if you're doing them properly, your legs will get a good workout, too.

And Mickey was all about doing the moves right, telling us to use low weights, or even just bars with no weights on them, to make sure we had good form before trying to lift a heavy load.

Telling a bunch of competitive men, most of whom make their living on Wall Street or as salesmen, to scale back their loads, focus on form, and not pay any attention at all to how much the other guys were lifting is like telling Cub Scouts to not laugh at a fart joke. It simply doesn't work. It got pretty funny at times to see Dave looking over at Leo's bar before a workout, noticing that Leo had twenty pounds more on than Dave did, and scrambling to add two ten-pound bumper plates to his own. And if doing a lift with less than perfect technique was the only way they could move the weight, well, then what difference did it make. They still got the weights up over their heads, right?

The truth was that I didn't care how much those guys were lifting. I cared only that I was able to do it properly, and that I didn't hurt myself. The fear of injury haunted me, not because I felt that lifting was inherently dangerous, but because, as the months went by, I came to look forward to it more than any other part of the WOD. Being injured would mean I wouldn't be able to lift, and that simply wasn't an option. My father-in-law says he could never be an alcoholic because he likes drinking too much to ever give it up. I felt that way about lifting. The fifteen minutes or so we spent lifting, from 5:40 a.m. or so until 5:55 or 6 came to be my turn to shine. My focus on the form meant that my weights were increasing quickly. It became a self-fulfilling cycle. The more weight I lifted, the more I wanted to lift. And the more I lifted, the better I felt. While some of the other guys nursed injuries brought on by bad form, I stayed healthy. Sore, yes, but healthy. And although my personal bests on the lifts weren't the highest ones on the massive "best board" that loomed over the Annex floor, they were pretty high up there. I was still playing in the house league, but when it came to lifting, the other guys were the Hatfields on ice skates.

My body adapted. As I warmed up one morning in front of the Annex's mirrors, it dawned on me: I had muscles. I had always had strong legs from cycling, but the lifting had given me bulk where I had never had it: my shoulders, my chest, my arms. I wasn't carved, or ripped, but I was beefy. Favorite T-shirts no longer fit me; after another few months, it became embarrassing to be seen in my Timberland Mountain Athletics large T-shirt, a sentimental old favorite, or a "Got Mana?" tee I had picked up in Hawaii and become attached to over the years because washing still couldn't remove the lovely smell of sunscreen, as evocative a scent as I know. For the first time, my eyes weren't drawn immediately to my midsection to see just how husky I was. My eyes would eventually get there, but only after I had looked at my upper body first and approved.

So I bought new, extra-large T-shirts, and preened a little when people told me I was looking buff. It was one thing to hear it from a neighbor, at a college reunion, or from someone at work, but it meant a whole lot more to hear it from the 5:30 guys. One morning, after he had been trotting the globe for his job, Dave walked in and looked at me doing overhead presses. "Holy shit you're getting big, bro," he said. It should have been as simple as a nice thing to hear from another middle-aged man. But it may as well have been Billy Hatfield admitting I could skate better than he could. And if Dave thought I was getting bigger, could a muscle-up or a kip be far behind?

Still, the early-morning workouts were killing me. They required me to go to bed before my three school-age kids, and the early hour left me so tired when I got home after work it was hard to stay awake to help with homework. Training is a supremely selfish act. If there were a way to train and make it a little easier on everyone at home, I needed to look for it.

So when an "official" CrossFit box opened in Morristown, slightly farther away than the Annex, but offering evening and weekend classes, I reluctantly switched boxes. It didn't bother me at all that the Annex wasn't a CrossFit affiliate. Mickey had multiple degrees in training and kinesiology and I knew from my own experience that the cert course, while informative, wasn't exactly rigorous. There was no test to certify that we had paid attention, and a couple of weeks later I received my CrossFit Level 1 certification in the mail. (CrossFit has since changed the requirements for Level 1 certification. In order to be certified, coaches have to pass a 55-question written test, and be recertified every five years. So while I officially attended the cert, I am no longer a certified Level 1 trainer.)

CrossFit Morristown was just a few miles from the Morristown National Historic Park, which commemorates the 1779–80 winter encampment of the Continental Army. Detailed records aren't available, but some climatologists will tell you that 1779–80 was the coldest winter ever recorded in New Jersey. CrossFit Morristown seemed like a good place to suffer.

Built in what looked to be a former automobile dealership, the box was filled with weights, tires for flipping, and bars for pulling up. Stairs just inside the sliding garage-style door led to a loft with couches and a big TV. It felt cool, kind of like a clubhouse. More like a purely CrossFit gym and less like a general training facility, the way the Annex did.

It was also populated almost entirely with people way, way younger than me. Nobody else at the box had gray hair, and as far as I could tell, nobody else was ever in a rush to get out of the WOD to get home to help the kids with their social studies homework. I was used to working out with guys my own age. They could kick my ass just as well as the youngsters at CrossFit Morristown. But my peers never called me sir, the way the young woman behind the counter often did when I'd check in.

Still, there was an enthusiasm and vibrancy to the place at 6 p.m. on a weeknight or 10 a.m. on Saturday that the Annex lacked at 5:30 in the morning. The music had been recorded after 1985, for one thing, and ran the spectrum from rap to metal to ska and Celtic punk like the Dropkick Murphys; the Annex's music selection, early in the morning at least, was frozen in the Reagan administration. And there was far more chatter at these classes than there ever was predawn at the Annex. For another, the athletes at Morristown were always talking about their social lives, which seemed to revolve around the box. During warm-ups, there was always a lot of talk about who was hooking up with whom, as well as what kind of booze you could have while still on the Paleo Diet.

It helped also that the owner and head instructor was drop-dead gorgeous and the most complete CrossFit athlete I'd ever seen. Karianne could do things on pull-up bars, with rings, and with Olympic weight bars that I'd never seen anybody do, not even the hardbodies at the cert. She had also assembled a cast of coaches—Mike, Leo, Jared—who made getting your ass kicked seem like the most fun thing in the world. I was a regular at CrossFit Morristown for a few months, but I never truly felt a part of the community. Rather, I felt like the uncle who had dropped in on a favorite nephew at college for a visit. It was fun, but I knew I didn't really belong there. I went back to the Annex, and I stayed there. For good.

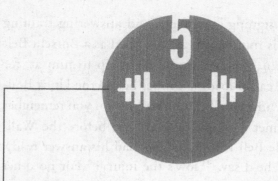

# A Few Words About Pain, Fatigue, and Nausea

The great American marathoner Bill Rodgers, who won both the New York City Marathon as well as the Boston Marathon four times each between 1975 and 1980, was a regular on the pre-race pasta dinner circuit, and had a well-deserved reputation as a man of the people for patiently signing autographs and answering training questions. His routine was as well oiled as a Borscht Belt comic's. When someone would come up to him at, for example, the carbo-loading dinner before the Utica Boilermaker 15K and say, "Bill, I don't know if you remember me, but we met a couple of years ago before the Wallingford Jingle Bell Run," Rodgers had his answer ready. "Sure, sure," he'd say. "How's the injury?" For no other answer could be as correct as "How's the injury?" It was axiomatic at the dawn of the running boom and remains axiomatic today, some forty years later, that if you run often enough, you will eventually get an injury that affects your performance.

Rodgers's device works equally well for CrossFit. As I write this, I am aware of a pain and fatigue in my arms and deltoids brought on by, in general, five consecutive days of WODs and, in particular, by yesterday's Olympic weight-lifting session featuring bent-over rows. I am also aware and perhaps slightly alarmed by a persistent and long-running dull ache in both knees that I can't help but think has something to do with an activity as benign as jumping rope.

Oh, and right above my left elbow, something is really sore. It hurts like hell, a sharp, what-the-fuck kind of pain that shoots like electricity as soon as I grab a rope to climb or grip a bar to do a pull-up. This pain is different from the pain of muscular soreness, which you have to expect with training like CrossFit. This pain means something is way wrong and needs to be addressed. Knowing the difference is a key to survival in this world. I need to get it checked.

Pain, soreness, fatigue, and even nausea are a regular part of any type of intense athletic training. In a weird way, pain and fatigue are signs that the training is working, that muscles and lung capacity are growing as you push yourself. But they are so central to the culture of CrossFit that when Uncle Pukie appears at a WOD, it is generally taken as a good sign, a sign that an athlete is working so damn hard that she has driven herself to exercise-induced nausea, puking outside the door of the box or into a strategically placed trash can.

Unless you're the puker. Then all it does is suck.

Another favorite T-shirt character, the short-armed T. Rex, celebrates the fact that athletes have pushed themselves so far that their arms feel as if they have become the tiny appendages the most fearsome of creatures is destined to not be able to use in his effort to rule the jungle.

This, to me, is the characteristic that best defines Cross-Fit. I've been part of a lot of different athletic subcultures, from swimming to cycling to mountaineering. They all in one way or another celebrate the fact that they train hard, and long, and challenge themselves with crazy races and events and stunts. Climb every peak over ten thousand feet in the Lower 48? Sure. Ride from Boston to Montreal and back without stopping for sleep? Of course. I know people who, if their houses were on fire, would on the way to the door grab their "I Survived the Shawangunks" T-shirt so that the world knew they had finished a particularly grueling triathlon, rather than take treasured family heirlooms like photo albums or Grandpa's framed citizenship documents.

But none wear pushing yourself to the point of puking, then going back to finish the workout, with the same pride as CrossFit athletes. What seems just plain fucking crazy to the rest of the world is a huge badge of honor to CrossFitters. Exercise-induced nausea has a variety of causes, and, according to experts, has nothing to do with what kind of shape you're in. An athlete training for the Olympics can be just as susceptible to hurling during a hard workout as a suburban dad trying to get back into shape after five years of couch surfing. Causes vary, from starting the workout with low blood sugar, as is often the case during early morning workouts, to motion sickness from all the contents of your belly being jostled around, to nerves, to restricted blood flow to the stomach to dehydration to overhydration.

I wear my Pukie the Clown T-shirt with excellent pride.

But I'm a puker from way back. When my eighth-grade gym class ran a mile every Friday immediately after a lunch of half-cooked pepperoni pizza and grape-ade, I would typically finish in the top three, then promptly step to the side of the instructor and deposit that lunch on the weed-choked grass of the William J. Galvin Middle School's lawn. I figured it was a small price to pay for being fast. I had been slow for so long that I would have given blood to finish in the top three. For four years as a high school sprinter, I deposited the slim remains of my high school lunch on the grass infields of tracks all across eastern Massachusetts after running for less than a minute in the 440-yard dash. One particular trash can at Boston's Commonwealth Armory was my go-to stop after the 300-yard dash during indoor track season. My teammates were so accustomed—and unalarmed—to seeing me heave and heave again after the races that they'd pat me on the back, mid-barf, with a "Nice race, Steve-o." It didn't matter. I could routinely finish in the top three in these races, and sometimes even win.

These incidents all occurred right after races, though, which means that nerves probably played a large part. I wrapped myself up so tight getting ready to run that it was a wonder I didn't puke *before* the race, as lots of athletes are known to do. Eliminating the contents of my gut before a race didn't help. I tried it once and ended up dry-heaving over the barrel. Skipping lunch on the day of meets didn't help, and would only leave me weak with hunger. Still, to this day, I associate the smell of puke with track meets just as closely as I do Ben-Gay and body funk.

Once I grew up, though, I figured my puking days were over. As an adult, I no longer worked my anaerobic system so hard that lunch would want to come up, I could pretty much work out when I wanted to, and I had ceased to get very nervous about how I was going to do in a race, knowing that the mantle of champion of the Chatham Fishawack Festival four-miler was beyond my grasp. (Of course, there was the time I ran it with a bottle and a half of excellent Oregon pinot noir still being filtered by my kidneys, and I deposited it so violently by the side of the road just fifty yards from the finish line that the Chatham Emergency Squad came running with oxygen and a stretcher, as if my ego needed oxygen and a ride. But that was an aberration.)

Then I started CrossFit.

The first time I booted should not have come as a surprise, for I had been forewarned, although that didn't occur to me until later. It was during my time among the youth at CrossFit Morristown. It was the day after Christmas, a Christmas I had spent enjoying some good wine and a lot of good food. The WOD was planned almost as if the coaches had known we had been bad the day before and were due for some penance. They delivered. Immediately across the street from the box was a steep hill, up which ran Ann Street. We were each to pair up with an athlete of similar weight, and we were to take turns carrying each other up and down the hill, all the way to the traffic light at the top, a total of ten times. I paired up with Brian, the only other guy in the place who looked to be over thirty-five. (I was wrong; he was thirty-two, but had a one-month-old at home, which would age anyone prematurely.)

Then we talked, awkwardly, about how we were going to do this. For someone who's in decent shape, carrying an adult, who in this case said he was a 180-pound man and a total stranger, is an act whose intimacy far outweighs its intensity. There's no way to do it, no hold, no grip, that doesn't present—especially to a sophomoric mind like mine—some sort of sexual overtone. Care to hop on my back? How about my shoulders, so I can have your junk pressed against the back of my head? In my arms, like I'm carrying you newlywed-style across a threshold?

We settled on the classic firemen's carry, in which I would squat down in front of Brian, he would drape himself across me with his belly pressed squarely into my right shoulder. He'd wrap one arm around my left side and I'd grab his wrist with my left hand and balance him with my right.

I was in trouble from the start. Everything was conspiring against me. Plain and simple, I was hungover as hell. A couple of pre-WOD espressos hadn't helped, a lesson it would take me years to learn. Brian's claim to weigh 180 was as much of a whopper as his sweaty ass, which was way too close to my face for comfort. And holy shit was Ann Street steep.

But we made it to the top, each of us huffing, me from the exertion and Brian from the jostling against my shoulder, which forced air from his lungs as if he were a bellows,

We got back down much more quickly, of course, despite the icy footing.

"Sorry for the bouncing, dude," I said as I put him down on Bank Street. "Only nineteen more to go." A wave of nausea was starting to rise. Not just in my stomach, but in my legs and arms, as if the acid churning in my belly had somehow found its way into my muscles. This isn't good, I thought, trying to think good thoughts, of fresh breezes and clean air and cute puppies. . . .

"Get on," Brian commanded, squatting down so I could lower myself. As I did, he rose, eager to get up the hill, and driving his shoulder into my rigorously ambiguous stomach. With each step he took up the hill, his shoulder drove into my belly, compressing my stomach and sending the acid farther out into the distant outposts of my body. The breezes I was thinking of started to blow, fetid and stinky. The air, no longer clean, had blown all the way from a third-world city, and the puppy had diarrhea. It took a lot of thought about *not puking* to keep it in. But I did.

Up and down. Two down. Brian was eager to hop back on but I asked for a minute to compose myself as I breathed out as hard as I could. One of the keys to beating exercise-induced nausea is to rid the body of as much carbon dioxide, a by-product of exertion, by exhaling as hard as you can by blowing out of your mouth. (It's an old trick used by mountaineers, called pressure breathing, in which they force themselves to exhale rather than gulp air, which every cell in the body is screaming for.) I pushed breath out, steam rising in the cold air as I tried to think of something besides the bile rising in my throat. Brian stood by, watching the other teams get ahead of us, then lap us. He looked down at the ice, hands on hips, idly kicking at a piece of ice.

"Get on," I said, then hoisted him up as I lurched up the hill. His weight had doubled since the last trip and my legs seemed to have lost their communication link with the rest of my body. While other teams buzzed around us, up and down the hill, I started up at a lurch, a slow walk. Brian talked me through it, urging me through my pauses. I would look up the hill and choose a marker, like a light post, and make it a goal to reach it without stopping. It worked a couple of times, but as I struggled to keep up with the other teams, my efforts resulted in more feelings of nausea rather than any forward progress. Sweat burst from my forehead, my scalp, my chest. I tried to suck in the cold air to dowse the fire burning in my gut, but the fire was spreading too quickly. I put Brian down about ten yards from the top. I moved off into a small parking alcove, and I retched. And retched. And sweat. But mostly I retched. Brian stood by, embarrassed, it would seem, not that his lame partner was booting into the dirty snow and ice in a Morristown parking lot, but more because this loser was causing him to miss his workout.

I was done for the day. There was no amount of scaling

down or substituting another WOD that could make me keep going. Disgusted with myself, I shuffled back to the box and ascended the stairs to a small lair that housed a few beat-up sofas and chairs in front of a giant TV. I plopped down and thought about a conversation I had had in this very spot with a guy who had just finished his WOD. He was raving about the benefits and effects of CrossFit. "I've lost fifteen fucking pounds!" he crowed. "My shirts don't fit me anymore. I'm crushing my pickup basketball game."

"Awesome," I said, looking over his shoulder as if I had been trapped at a party by a Ben Franklin impersonator.

"There's just one thing. Never, ever drink the night before a workout."

That got my attention. "Never? Nothing? Not even a beer?"

"Well, if you can stop at one beer, you should be fine. But don't ever come here hungover."

I wished I had remembered this conversation about an hour ago. Lesson learned.

Add to that list: never come caffeinated. I've never had a problem dropping a double shot of espresso before hopping on my bike or heading to the pool. In fact, coffee is so engrained in cycling culture that most cycling clubs feature "coffee shop rides," routes that begin, end, and pause at coffee shops or cafés for refueling. So I figured that, if I were going to expect myself to get my ass out of bed most mornings at five to get to the Annex, I would need a double shot of my dark master.

I figured wrong. Way wrong. Whether it was the acid of the coffee, or taking it on an empty stomach, or just the plain exertion of the drill, Pukie came to visit me not too long after I returned to the Annex. Mickey was coaching one early morning. Nothing felt right to me. I hadn't slept well, I felt spastic, and my head wasn't in the game. It wasn't Mickey's fault, of course. I was the dumb-ass who had pounded two shots as an eye opener before embarking on a course of thrusters and double unders well before sunrise.

But he didn't help, either. I felt both his stare drilling through me and the familiar wildfire taking off in my belly and throat, of bile rising with each thruster, of barely digested coffee mixing with stomach acids to form a witch's brew of disgust that wanted to do nothing but leave my stomach.

Try as I might, the brew won the fight against gravity. This time, conditioned by my experience on Ann Street, I made it to the barrel near where Mickey was standing, arms crossed, impassive. I heaved. He stood. I heaved some more and still he stood. I wasn't expecting a sorority-sister-holding-my-hair-back kind of moment, not at a place where Metallica's *Kill 'Em All* blared before sunrise, but I thought I'd get more than "Make sure you wipe down the edges of that barrel." I did.

And then I did something that surprised even me. After rinsing my mouth with cold water, and absorbing the condescendingly sympathetic glimpses of my class-mates, many of whom had by now finished the WOD, I went back to the puddle of sweat that marked my work-station, grabbed my kettle bell, and finished the workout. Getting sick was a weakness, one that I could eliminate by learning from the experience and chipping away at the flaws that made it happen. I was eight minutes slower than everyone else that class, but I was the only one who got a "right on" along with the usual post-WOD fist bump from Mickey.

That morning, puking wasn't the badge of honor. Getting back up and finishing was.

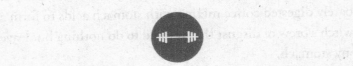

One of the keys to survive—and thrive—in CrossFit is learning how to tell the difference between regular old soreness brought on by hard exercise, and the kind of pain that's telling you something is way, way wrong, or at least wrong enough to become way, way wrong if left unattended. Trap your hand between a dumbbell and the floor, as I once saw someone do, and you'll crush bone and rend skin in a way that draws blood. That's obviously way wrong. But what if you feel a twinge in your shoulder after working on muscle-ups? You've been trying to defy gravity by swinging yourself up into a hand press in the air for the last thirty minutes. Of course your shoulder hurts. But will it go away by itself, or should you run to the doctor or physical therapist to have it looked at?

Most important of all: can I work out tomorrow?

There are two types of muscular soreness. When you're in the middle of a workout, going hard, your muscles start to burn because they're producing lactic acid (LA). Pause for a minute, or back off the intensity, and the burn will subside. Part of the point of training is to push back the time of arrival of lactic acid, and to adapt to its presence so it doesn't cause you to stop. Once the workout is over, LA clears the system within an hour or so, and a good cooldown will ensure that it's flushed from your body.

The second type of pain is delayed onset muscle soreness (DOMS), the result of tiny tears in the muscle—or, more specifically, between the muscles and surrounding tissue. These tears release chemicals that cause swelling, and it's that swelling that makes you sore. DOMS is the reason people can walk normally immediately after crossing the finish line of a marathon, limp the next day, and can't get out of a chair the day after that. It's why Cross-Fitters can put on their sweatshirts after a WOD and drive home but can't control a coffee cup or a computer mouse that afternoon. It's most likely to occur when you start a new exercise program or mix it up some way. If you do the same thing all the time, your muscles adapt and you won't feel the soreness of micro tears, just the ache of lactic acid, and not even that if you don't push yourself hard enough.

But if your routine is anything but routine, if it is "constantly varied," then it stands to reason that you will be constantly sore. Welcome to CrossFit.

This is where experience comes in handy. I've enjoyed a lifetime of physical activity that has included training regimens in swimming, running, cycling, triathlons, mountaineering, and rowing. Over the years, I've had sore arms, sore legs, sore necks, hips, backs, knees, and elbows. My soma has been sore, and my soul has been sore. But I've figured out the difference between the workaday aches caused by training and the deep-muscle fatigue caused by maximum efforts like racing, and the I-think-I-just-separated-my-shoulder moment of a trauma. I've always been able to loosen up in the days after a tough workout by moving slowly but surely in the hope that my muscles would unwork themselves. One way or another, the idea was to get back to training, even if it meant a bit of rest and the sometime obligatory ice packs and ibuprofen. The older I get, the better able I am to judge how much rest and recuperation I need.

Unlike my behavior in most of my other athletic incarnations, I have taken very much to heart CrossFit's admonition about warming up vigorously, cooling down with caution, and considering mobility a part of my daily routine, not just something to do, idly, sometimes, as I was standing around waiting for the activity to start. There are days when the longest part of a CrossFit workout is spent urging your muscles into just a centimeter more of give. It can be a strange sight, and a shock to a newcomer.

CrossFit boxes come equipped with foam and plastic cylinders in a variety of lengths, diameters, and firmness; lacrosse balls, sometimes taped together to form a sort of scrotal sack; giant rubber bands of varying, color-coded tensions; lengths of rope, broomsticks, dowels, and pieces of PVC pipe. All are designed to help you work kinks out of your muscles, joints, and tendons, and to get ready to go back into the fray. It is perfectly normal to see CrossFitters astride those cylinders, rolling their asses on the hard foam to work out the kinks from yesterday's walking lunges. The lacrosse ball sack is run down the muscle pads on either side of the spine, while a single lax ball can be driven into muscle just about anywhere, at any time. (I'm sitting in my office chair right now as I write this, massaging a lacrosse ball deep into my calves in between paragraphs.) We wrap the rubber bands around our feet and pull back with our arms to urge our legs into a millimeter more of a stretch than the day before. We hold the broomsticks in a wide grip and run them up, over, and behind our torsos—a pass-through—to make our shoulders and chests more flexible. Then we hold it up over our heads and squat down, deeply, chest and shoulders up, and hold that bar way overhead until our quads scream and our hip flexors surrender to our will.

We co-opt the best bits of yoga into our mobility routines, facing doglike downward and then upward to loosen and strengthen pretty much everything. We push one leg behind us, cross the other in front, and lower to the floor in pigeon pose, lengthening quadriceps and hips. We prostrate ourselves in child's pose to a god whose blessing will allow us to do one more burpee in the time allotted than we did when last we faced this particular WOD. We stand, backs, butts, arms, and heels flush against the wall, and slide our arms up and over our heads, which is much harder than it sounds.

Some of us sit, after workouts, in tubs filled with ice to stop muscular swelling. We take post-WOD contrast showers, dousing ourselves with ice-cold water to quell the swelling before returning to warmer water, a process we repeat over and over again after workouts as if we were annealing newly forged metal. Because, in fact, we are.

Why? There is not a single study in scientific literature that can claim to prove, with evidence, that stretching works. But neither is there one that proves it doesn't. Most come to the conclusion that we should do it anyway, scientific proof be damned. But as anybody who ever paid attention will tell you, the more fluid and supple and stretchy we are, the better our form will be. And the better our form, the more weight we can move. The more reps we can get in, the farther and faster and harder we can run and row and cycle and swim. We can be better. Good form solves all problems. Most important, good form prevents injury.

Maybe that's why I've never had the kind of injury that leads people to go up to Bill Rodgers at a spaghetti dinner and ask for advice about the pain in their arch. For whatever reason, I was blessed with the body of a workhorse—or, more to the point, a plowhorse. Nothing fast. Nothing pretty. But durable. When other runners complained of knee injuries, I listened sympathetically but didn't understand. When my swim lane mates had to take weeks or months out of the pool to nurse sore shoulders, I missed them, and swam on. When cycling friends would complain of wrist, neck, shoulder, or knee soreness that made cycling impossible, I'd check my saddle height to make sure it was correct, and throw a leg over.

I had always paid attention to correct form, no matter what I was doing. Not because I wanted to look good, but because I needed every advantage I could muster to be able to keep up. Turns out that not blindly thrashing my arms was helping me swim faster, but it was also protecting my shoulders and hips. Taking the time to set up my bike in a way to maximize both comfort and speed allowed me to put in a lot of miles without having to visit a chiropractor.

All of which served me very well when I started doing CrossFit, which emphasizes technique over all things, as well it should. It's one thing to half-ass a sit-up. But try to fake your way through a complicated Olympic lift like a hanging squat snatch and the results can be catastrophic as 135 pounds come crashing down on your head and neck.

That's why On Ramp is a standard CrossFit protocol. Designed to teach newcomers the basics of movements and terminology, On Ramp is an eight-class prerequisite to being able to attend a regular CrossFit WOD. Trained instructors use those same broomsticks we use for pass-throughs as stand-ins for barbells, and teach the foundations of each movement. This is where you learn to keep your weight on your heels when you squat so that you can wiggle your toes when you're butt is near the ground, and so that your chest and shoulders stay up. On Ramp is where you learn to shrug your shoulders when you clean a bar, push your elbows up and through when you front-squat, and always squeeze your butt cheeks together when you're at the top of a move so you know your hips are fully extended.

This is also where you learn you have zero flexibility, aren't nearly as strong as you think you are, and may be able to run for two hours at a steady trot but can't go more than ninety seconds flat-out. It's also where you learn where you excel beyond your peers, be it at things involving leg strength or the ability to hold a plank pose. And you will pray for these exercises to be programmed every day so that you can grasp the opportunity, no matter how fleeting, to feel smug.

But pay attention and do it right. Because if you don't, you will get hurt. And do it right, even when you're well into a workout and starting to get tired. Especially when you're tired.

But aren't we always tired?

CrossFit suggests that you WOD no more than three days in a row. Not that you do nothing on that rest day. You work on your mobility, you go for a walk, maybe throw a Frisbee around. But you don't WOD. Not even a little bit. You can then start it up again after a day of rest. So if the week starts with a workout on Monday, then Tuesday and Wednesday, you can rest Thursday, then work out Friday through Sunday. That's six WODs in seven days. Lots of exercise.

There are those among us who pay no attention to this rule, and they tend to be the same ones who nurse chronic injuries, who show up at the box slowly rotating a shoulder with a wince and a troubled look. For in the same way that a sore, swollen muscle responds to the cold packs, a tired body responds to rest. When you exercise, you expend energy. When you exercise a lot, or very intensely, you expend a lot of energy. Replace the energy with the proper nourishment, fluids, and sleep and you will recover. Skip any part of the process and you won't recover fully. It sounds obvious, but laying off, lying low, lying around is as important to progress as WODing. As the old cycling saw goes: you get fast in bed.

This was yet another lesson I learned the hard way, in August 2013, when in a burst of enthusiasm I dug myself a hole so deep over the course of a week that I then spent another week climbing out of it. When I look at my training notes for that time now, I wonder what the hell I was thinking. With such entries as "felt bone-tired, depleted," "felt shitty," and "terrible night's sleep," you'd think I would have known to back off. But I didn't. Starting Sunday, August 18, and running through Saturday, August 31, I worked out eleven times, including a pretty tough four-mile obstacle course race, and either walked or rode one of New York City's public bikes, a Citi Bike, the 2.8-mile round-trip between my office and Penn Station, New York, every workday. I also got up most mornings at five. There were just two consecutive days in there when I did absolutely nothing.

It all came to a head on Saturday the thirty-first. The Annex had planned to honor the nineteen Granite Mountain Hotshot forest fire fighters who had died at Yarnell, Arizona, in June 2013 by joining a national WOD that raised money for the dead men's families. "Hotshots 19" called for us to do a staggering six rounds of the following: 30 air squats to a medicine ball, 19 cleans of an 85-pound load, 7 pull-ups, and a 400-meter run. That's a total of 180 air squats, 114 cleans, 42 pull-ups, and 1.5 miles of running. As fast as you can. It's a lot.

Especially considering the volume of work I had done in the previous two weeks, and considering that the evening before I had been so exhausted I couldn't carry on a conversation and could only lie by the pool in a lounge chair drinking Budweiser Tall Boys. What's worse, a duvet of August humidity lay over New Jersey, and I should have been smarter and cut my losses by just staying in bed. Clearly, my body was telling me it was time to rest. And I wasn't listening.

We were leaving for a week's vacation in Quebec that afternoon, a week in which I was sure to hike and swim but not sure to WOD, so I wanted to get in one more burner. Besides, doing Hotshots 19 had been my idea; I was the one who pushed Mickey to program it, despite his better judgment that it was too much volume. "We should honor these guys," I told him, and said as much in an email I sent to everyone at the box.

I knew, from the moment I put my bare foot on the floor to get out of bed, that the day was not going to go well. Neither my mind nor my body was ready to do Hotshots 19 and honor the guys who had died. I was tired in my bones. My mind was blank and wrung out. I couldn't focus on the warm-up, which despite its easy pace had my heart rate soaring, a sure sign of overtraining. Sweat flowed too easily. "I got this," I told myself. But I didn't believe it.

Six people showed up for the WOD. Under normal conditions, I would be a mid-packer on this one. Squats were never a problem; nor were cleans, although 19 per round was a lot of throwing around. Pull-ups still sucked for me, but that was nothing new. Running 400s? Always dicey. Short enough to want to make you go hard, long enough to make you suffer. The 400 course at the Annex was an out-and-back on River Road, slightly uphill to the turnaround point marked with a spray-painted CROSSFIT on the pavement in front of the door to a school bus company.

Mickey stood, his usual morning statue, and counted down the start. "Three, two, one, GO!" I knocked out the squats, finished the pull-ups with the help of a band, making note of the utter lack of power in my arms, then set to the cleans. I should have been able to do them in a single set of ten, caught my breath, then finished them with a set of nine, but found myself right away settling on three sets of five and one of four. Rather than putting the bar back on the ground with control, I dropped it as soon as I had completed the lift. That was a very bad sign.

It was about to get worse. I headed out the door to start the run right where I thought I'd be, in the middle of the pack, behind a new, fast guy named Mark, the aerobic freak Jason, and Anne. I may as well have been running up a ski jump. My legs had no give, no turnover. Before I had gone fifty yards, Lisa, a good runner who can't do pull-ups because of a shoulder injury, passed me. That's okay, I thought to myself. She didn't do the pull-ups. I'm doing more work. This sucks, but I can do it.

That's when Chris Duignan passed me. Duignan, a former collegiate rower and marine, was easily the most affable person at the Annex. As funny and self-deprecating as he was eager to learn the ropes, Chris threw himself into workouts with an enthusiasm that far outstripped his conditioning, flexibility, or strength. He climbed ropes with such vigor that the telltale burn on his ankle from bracing himself on the ascent became infected. He sweat so vigorously, even after he'd finished the WOD, showered, and toweled off, that he'd say the shower "didn't take." The standard line on Chris, one on which he agreed, was that when he lost twenty or thirty pounds he was going to be an animal. You could see it when he rowed and his experience in a collegiate boat showed.

But none of that showed when he ran. When he passed me and then offered a "Come on now" as encouragement, I felt as if I had been gut-shot. Fuck. Duignan's passing me? How can this be? He left a spray of sweat in his wake. I sped up, struggling to maintain contact. I caught up, moved in just behind his shoulder, and matched his pace.

For about five strides.

I was now, officially, in last place. And we were only finishing the first round. I told myself that it was okay, I'd be okay, that the others couldn't possibly hold this pace, not with this oppressive humidity, that my workhorse nature would help me grind it down. I didn't believe a word of it, but I said it to myself, hoping that if I said it enough it would become true. I had every reason in the world not to be performing well. Every single sign had foretold that

I was overtrained and didn't belong there, that the right thing to do was to have stayed in bed. Nonetheless, there was that old feeling all over again: I was fat and slow. All talk and show, no go.

The second round picked up with the air squats, an exercise I can usually do all day long. But not today. Rather than pumping them out unbroken—thirty in a row, without pause—I broke them into groups of ten. Take a big problem and make it a few small ones. It was as if sections of rebar had been put in my quads. They simply wouldn't bend. My energy was low, fuel seemingly nonexistent. And my will? I had none.

Mickey scowled. Duignan sweated. Anne and Lisa and Jason and Mark ran and cleaned and pulled up. I paced in place, trying to find a rhythm, a gear, some fuel, anything to get me going. But the fact was simple, and unavoidable. I was tapped out.

I used to swim for a coach who from time to time would come over to a swimmer during warm-ups and say, "Climb on out of there. Why don't you go get a pizza or something? It's just not happening for you today. You're struggling." The couple of times I got such a tap, he was dead on right. Here's the thing about CrossFit: nobody will ever say that to you. If you started, you're gonna finish. An obvious trauma like a dislocated shoulder gets you out of that, but being tired or feeling tapped out or even having bloody palms from too many pull-ups is no excuse, if for no other reason than that you are training your mind to be as tough as your body.

So I took twenty pounds off the bar and cleaned 65 pounds rather than the 85 I had started with. I switched the white elastic pull-up band to the super-strength black one, and I shuffled through the 400s as if I were carrying a load far heavier than mere fatigue.

When I came in after completing the fourth round, I checked my time on the digital stopwatch on the wall. It read 30:00 exactly. It seemed like a good place to stop. Thirty minutes is a good long time to exercise hard, it was my fifth workout of the week, vacation was about to start, and I had done my part to honor the memory of the fallen firefighters. So I ambled over to the bench where a dry T-shirt awaited me while the others chipped away at their sixth round.

"What are you doing?" Mickey asked as I stripped off my soaking workout shirt.

"I'm done."

"No, you have two more rounds to go," he said.

"I'm fried. Been a long week. I'm finished."

Mickey is twenty years younger than I am. I'm much farther along my path than he is. I'd like to think that as an elder, I had some respect coming to me. I'd like to think that over the past year or so, a year of grinding it out, of pushing and lifting and collapsing on the stinking turf after depleting myself, after puking and still finishing

WODs, I had enough cred to be able to bounce a check to the boss once in a while.

I also like to think I will never again see the look that flashed through Mickey's eyes, just for a second, when he realized I was serious, that I really was quitting. I could tell he wanted to call me out, to say that Duignan and Lisa and my wife were still going, and to question not my manhood but my very sense of humanity, because who gets up on a Saturday morning in summer to do a workout like this to honor guys who didn't have the luxury of quitting, and then walks away with two rounds to go? What the fuck is wrong with you? he wanted to say.

But he didn't. He just turned his back on me and walked away, which was worse. I slunk off to the locker room while the others finished the workout. When they were done, nobody said a word to me. They chatted excitedly about how hard the workout was, how their strategies had changed as it went along, how they struggled but adapted and finished. Their smiles to me were polite, but it was clear that I wasn't one of them, because I hadn't done what I had set out to do, and they had.

And then this flashed through my head: What makes you think you can do this?

My God. What had I just done? I had chosen to listen to the voice, the old one, the ancient one, the one that told me I wasn't good enough, not as good as the others and that it was okay to quit, because I was really tired. What

94

had started out as shame turned to guilt and then horror as I realized what I had done. It wasn't just letting Duignan beat me. Or looking like a lesser man in Mickey's eyes. I had spent the better part of a year making the voice a little quieter each time I refused to stop. And now I had just let it back in the game. Because I was tired. Fuck.

I had proven to myself over much of the past year that I had the guts and the heart to lose control of my bodily functions and still complete the task at hand. I had earned the respect from people I revered. But I had thrown that all away in just the few seconds it took to make a bad decision. I had let my pain and fatigue overcome my willpower. It was a brutal way to relearn the lesson. You never quit a workout. Never. Don't get so tired—or sore, or sick—that you can't finish a job you start.

That was the last workout I ever quit.

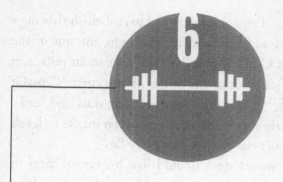

# Diet and Body Image

It's telling that a book about CrossFit would contain a seven-thousand-word chapter on fatigue, pain, and nausea and a chapter half that length on nutrition. Because while mountains of ever-changing information about diet and nutrition and their relationship to health and performance are published each year, the basic tenet of nutrition in the CrossFit world is one I've already mentioned: don't eat shitty food. If you absolutely had to embellish that nugget, you could add this: eat just the right amount of the good stuff. As CrossFit founder Greg Glassman puts it in the very first sentence of his brilliantly succinct "CrossFit in 100 Words," "Eat meat and vegetables, nuts and seeds, some fruit, little starch and no sugar. Keep intake to levels that will support exercise but not body fat."

These are words we all could live by, CrossFitters or not. Because whether you want to lose a few pounds to look good at a wedding or get all *Biggest Loser* to regain your life, nothing works like a calorie-restricted diet based on plant foods and lean proteins. This isn't anything new: high school wrestlers, body builders, models, actresses, and magazine editors with upcoming TV appearances have known for generations that if you need to drop a few pounds quickly, you stop eating carbs, be they processed, like pretzels, or even whole grain, like brown rice, and tuck into a limited amount of salmon, skinless chicken breast, kale, lettuce, and tomatoes—but not potatoes, bread, cereals, even carrots and apples. Take it easy on the salt and drink a ton of water. Maybe you use a little bit of olive oil and vinegar to add flavor, but nothing processed, and nothing with sugar. Just have to have a drink? Try red wine but stay way away from beer.

For someone who has spent a lifetime being traumatized by being a fat kid, you'd think I would have been more concerned about all this stuff. But when it comes to diet, I've always been way over in the liberal arts wing of the fitness world, approaching sports and my various workouts with a combination of rationalization and I'm-just-an-English-major ignorance. Exercise was all just part of a complete life. No need to get carried away by obsessing over my diet. Besides, I worked out so much, I could eat whatever I wanted, right? Those arguments work up until about age twenty-five; after that, I bought progressively larger pants and tried to not go too nuts with my bête noir: sweets.

When I went through my CrossFit certification class, I was shocked by how much time the instructors spent talking about diet. You'd lose weight, they told us, which would certainly make pull-ups easier, and you'd feel good, too. You would develop something we are all proud of but went largely unspoken: the CrossFit Body. Muscles, ripped and hard. CrossFitters spend a lot of time and effort developing their muscles, so it's little wonder that a whole lot of skin is visible in most boxes. It's perfectly acceptable for guys to rip off their shirts at the slightest exertion and do the WOD bare-chested (but not at the Annex, where the older male clientele would rather be waterboarded than take off the T-shirts they bought at a bar in the Virgin Islands on vacation ten years ago). Lululemon has prospered catering to female CrossFitters who want to cover only what they need to; sports bras and tight short-shorts are the norm (but again, not at the Annex, where the older female clients are more modest).

As I mentioned before, the Zone Diet, the brainchild of Dr. Barry Sears, held that any person, athlete or not, could achieve optimal performance with a diet whose caloric composition was 40 percent complex carbohydrates, 30 percent protein, and 30 percent fat. On the Zone, you could have a nice meal of, say, chicken with soba noodles and a couple of servings of vegetables. But in order to make the Zone work, you needed to weigh your food, especially in the first weeks of the program as you dialed in portion sizes.

This seemed like way too much work to me, and frankly, a bit of a buzzkill. I wanted to get in better shape, and sure, it would be great to shed a layer of fat to show off my new guns, but I'm a guy who doesn't see the need for kitchen cabinets when countertops hold plates and glasses just as well. Weighing my food seemed way too obsessive, if not just shy of lunatic fringe.

The Paleo Diet gets its name from the fact that you eat only food that a caveman could have found. What could you eat? Meat and fish, including bacon and ham. Pretty much any green vegetables, avocados, nuts, and certain kinds of berries. No melons or mangoes or bananas—too high a glycemic load in those fruits. (Apparently Paleolithic man hadn't made it to the tropics.) While I knew the diet didn't include Fritos or Dr Pepper, I was surprised to learn what else was on the taboo list: milk and any milk-based products; grains, including corn, rice, and oats; potatoes, bread, cereal, refined sugar, and coffee.

The plans had one key point in common. "Don't try to eat like this all the time," the instructor said. "You'll go crazy. It doesn't work. Allow yourself to cheat. Be good eighty percent of the time and you'll see results." He mentioned that a lot of people were rigorously strict from Sunday night to Friday at 5 p.m. and let their hair down on the weekend. By letting their hair down he meant they had some drinks, maybe ate a baguette, had a burger on an actual bun or a handful of M&Ms.

It would have all sounded completely nuts to me had it not been for the experience of my colleague João Correia. João and I had worked together at *Bicycling* magazine, where it was perfectly acceptable to conduct a business meeting while out on a ride. That meant donning bike clothes. Nobody looks good in bike clothes. They're built for comfort and function while on the bike; like most athletic apparel, they don't flatter anybody who's not a professional. Even though João could rip the legs off most of us on a ride, his ample girth puffed against his kit as if it were a sausage casing. Too much high life entertaining clients had left him sixty pounds over the weight he raced at thirteen years before, when he had been a promising young rider on the European junior circuit.

But when a client noticed the natural form and ability lurking beneath the insulation and challenged him to get in shape, João threw himself at the task, working with a trainer as well as a nutritionist, who told him to "eat like a caveman."

So he did, cutting out the pasta he loved so much, snacking on almonds and blackberries instead of panini, and skipping the sugar he usually put in his espresso. (I don't know a single person who ever accepted the Taliban-like edict to give up caffeine.) The diet, combined with his rigorous training, allowed João to drop the sixty pounds in just five months. The transformation was so profound that people who hadn't seen him in a while walked right by him without even recognizing him. And the same client helped João realize a dream of racing again professionally in Europe, a dream he thought had been lost to his weight gain.

After João's transformation, I asked him if people treated him differently now that he had returned to his racing weight, and if it bothered him. "It bothered me more when people who hadn't seen me in a few years as I put on the weight would say, 'João, is that you?' as if I had become a different person when I gained the weight. I was still the same guy. I just wasn't as fast."

It reminded me of something that happened when I was in my early thirties. I was swimming with the local YMCA masters team, and we went to the state championships, where I won five medals in my age group, and the team won more than twenty. The director of the Y was so proud of us that he took the team photo we had posed for on the pool deck after the meet and blew it up to poster size and mounted it just inside the door of the pool, for everyone to see.

There I was in all my pre-swim glory, in shorts and flip-flops and a pair of sunglasses and nothing else but the medals draped around my neck, my spare tire there for all to see. At the office one day, a woman I had worked with for three years came up to me and said with more of a sneer than she should have, "I saw your picture at the Y. Nice. I had no idea you were so . . . so . . ." The look on my face must have given her pause. "So, beefy."

It shouldn't have mattered. I knew I was beefy, or whatever other word she wanted to use. But her words killed me. They shouldn't have. I had just won five medals and swum two races faster than I ever had, before or since. But she wasn't seeing that. She was seeing the beef.

In a very gross simplification, both the Paleo and Zone diets work by jiggering hormones released by foods we eat. Certain foods can release a flood of insulin, which makes the body store fat while signaling the stomach to keep eating. (It's more than just an old advertising jingle that nobody can eat just one Lay's potato chip. The flood of insulin released by foods like chips only makes you want to eat more chips.) Sugar, in all its many forms, is one such food, as are processed carbohydrates and dairy foods. It's extremely counterintuitive, but the Paleo Diet holds that if you must have dairy, it should be heavy cream, and that you should stay as far away from "processed" skim milk as possible. The goal here is to eat only foods that don't mess up your hormonal balance by sending insulin coursing into your blood, but that do fill you up and make you feel satisfied. Vegetables and meat do this nicely; an apple can make you want to eat another apple. But eat that apple with some almonds and you should feel satisfied by the healthy fat dampening the insulin response.

It sounded easy. Eat this stuff, skip that stuff, and you'll lose weight. But when I surveyed my diet, I realized I was about to have my cheese moved in a pretty significant way. It's not as if I subsisted on fried chicken and lemonade, but I ate bread at every meal, loved cookies and pasta, and drank skim milk every morning. Among my ex-wife's many parting words to me were "I hope you find someone who will be sure to bring vegetables into your life, because I'm sure you won't find them on your own." I could live without soda and salty snacks and ice cream, but I had a drawer of candy in my office, and drank at least one beer or glass of wine every night, sometimes more. When you start reading labels, you realize: sugar is in everything we eat. Everything. Salad dressing. Condiments. Marinades. Yogurt. Cocktails.

During my time at CrossFit Morristown, the box sponsored a two-month nutrition challenge. I jumped right in.

We were given notebooks and told that we would write down every morsel of food and every drop of liquid we put in our mouths for the next month. Karianne, the box owner, would then review them and offer us advice on how to improve our performance. We were also given a list of approved foods, almost all of which were minimally processed, if processed at all. We were to be on the lookout for food with ingredients, especially sugar, and we were to eat things as close as possible to the form in which nature provided them. She advised us to empty our cupboards of all the bad foods she was sure were in there, as if Passover were about to start and we needed to get rid of leavened food. But I had decided I could suffer through this alone, and not subject my grade-school children to a life without pizza or Cheez-Its. The snacks and food might call out to me from their boxes and wrappers, but I would be strong. The stuff could stay.

Day one was a nightmare. Gone was my breakfast of a sandwich of almond butter on whole wheat toast, a glass of skim milk, and a glass of orange juice. In its place was three ounces of Canadian bacon, half a pint of raspberries, and a handful of almonds. That was at 7:30 a.m. By nine I was starving as I drove along Interstate 78 on my daily commute. I pulled into a Turkey Hill store, a sprawling emporium of snack foods, but not exactly a place filled with fresh fruits and lean meats. But if you look carefully, as I did, you'll find nuts, bottled water, and jerky.

I didn't want meat to become the center of my Paleo experience. I wanted to be the guy who did this all with salads and nuts, even though it rarely occurs to me to seek out vegetables on my own, although I dive right in when they're put in front of me. But I saw a bag of Oberto teriyaki jerky, and I pounced on it, knowing it would fill my belly well enough to get me to lunch. Plus, who doesn't love jerky?

I went on my usual lunchtime ride, a leisurely hour-long spin across flat Pennsylvania farmland, nothing too taxing. But my stomach growled as if I had just ridden all afternoon. Afterward, buying lunch in the cafeteria, I chose a chicken wrap with carrot sticks and bread-and-butter pickles rather than the chips or pretzels I usually got, and a bottle of sports drink to top off my fluid levels after the ride. That afternoon, as my coworkers celebrated someone's birthday with cupcakes, I stood with arms crossed and made polite refusal after polite refusal, even though the cupcakes were made by a woman who would later leave the company to open her own now-thriving bakery. Sugar was calling me, and I was trying not to hear.

That night, at the box, Karianne asked me how things were going. I told her about the breakfast and the jerky, and my lunch.

"What kind of wrap did you use for that sandwich?" she asked.

I told her it was a spinach tortilla.

106

"Skip it. It's poison," she said. "Same for the Gatorade. You don't need that for an hour ride. Water is fine. Bread-and-butter pickles are made with sugar. Lose them."

I had never heard something as seemingly wholesome as a spinach tortilla called poison, but then again I had never eaten Paleo.

That evening's dinner was half a roast chicken and a bag of spinach sautéed in olive oil. It wasn't too far from my usual dinner, lacking only some good rolls and a glass or two of wine. Later, rather than lying on the couch and enjoying a few M&Ms or pretzels as I usually did, I ate some almonds and drank several pints of water, then went to bed early, praying that sleep would deliver me from the desire to eat a box of Triscuits or a bag of Polly-O cheese sticks.

The next day wasn't any better. The wind was out of the west, a zephyr carrying the scent of the blooming onions cooking at Charlie Brown's, a local steak joint, and the garlic knots slowly baking at Hickory Pizza. Every desk in the office had doughnuts or Hershey Kisses on it, every meeting had cookies, every lunch had a mound of french fries served with it. But I stayed strong, ordering double portions of green beans and brisket to keep myself full. There were voices calling to me to eat. But there were voices calling to me at the gym, too, telling me to quit. I had learned to push them down, and I could push down the siren call of un-Paleo food, too.

Still, it took supreme acts of consciousness and will to stay on the program. Rather than just blindly accepting foods offered to me, like those tiny packets of snack mix on an airplane or samples at the supermarket, I learned to carefully consider what was being offered and to say no thank you if it wasn't Paleo. I carried around my own half-pound bag of smokehouse almonds, jerky, raw unsweetened coconut, and dried berries, figuring that if I became desperate and was faced with unhealthy, un-Paleo choices, I could always eat my own food. If my meal at a restaurant came with potatoes, I'd ask for a substitution of extra vegetables, or, if it was Saturday, a cheat day, take one bite of the mashed and enjoy. I opted out of the breadbasket and learned to stay on the perimeter of the supermarket, where the meat and vegetables are, the inner aisles being the pathway to processed sin. I drank only red wine, and only on Fridays, Saturdays, and Sundays, never during the week. Beer and I broke up. Like most breakups, it took a few times to truly take, and there were a few bouts of messy makeup sex. And I missed orange juice, with all its sugary tartness that could wake me up almost as well as a double espresso.

Breakfasts became an orgy of bacon as the microwave became coated with a film of pork fat. I put olive oil on everything because it was a very Paleo fat and helped make me feel full, and devoured bowls of gazpacho, not because the cavemen necessarily liked cold tomato soup, but because its minimal ingredients were all unprocessed. I learned to like oysters, a very Paleo food. My food was minimally processed if it had been processed at all. I skipped smoothies, because so many of them were based on fruit juices and yogurt, both verboten foods. My main cheat food was my mother-in-law's fresh chocolate chip cookies, which she baked only on Sundays and were gone, thanks to how fast they went at a big family dinner, by Sunday night. If I ordered a burger, I left the bun behind. I skipped cereals and rice.

Here's a page from my food diary for Monday, February 11:

---

Espresso, one at 8 a.m., one at 10 a.m.
Raspberries, almonds, and a chicken breast at 7 a.m.
Chicken breast, carrots, and celery at 12:30 p.m.
Tacos with grilled beef, turkey, cabbage, salsa, skipped the
   taco shell, 7 p.m.
8 almonds, 8 p.m.
120 ounces of water over the day

---

After a week, I had lost four pounds. After two weeks, seven. After a month, ten. After two months, twenty. I lost so much weight that I needed to buy new jeans. I texted Anne from the dressing room of a Levi's store: "I can fit in skinny jeans!" People commented, men and women, at my buffness. A colleague opened a meeting by saying, "Let's talk about how skinny Madden is." A friend's wife gave me a look that made me wonder if she were the real Mrs. Robinson. I preened. And my WODs started to improve, especially anything involving pull-ups or running, because I had just dropped 10 percent of my body weight. Imagine doing all these exercises with a twenty-pound dumbbell in your pocket, then imagine taking it out. Yes, you'd be faster. And yes, people would notice. And yes, they'd say something you wanted to hear.

No wonder people get so obsessed with this, I thought.

I really and truly felt, for the first time in my life, that I wasn't the fat kid in the class. I thought of my parents. Dad teasing my mother for her hamburger—no bun—served with tomatoes, lettuce, and cottage cheese while he enjoyed his Scotch and burgers served with beans and pan-fried new potatoes from a can, one of his specialties. Ma was pretty Paleo before the term had been coined.

I wasn't always good. On vacation in St. John, I fell hard off the wagon after a 3.5-mile swim, gorging myself on Double Stuf Oreos and Swedish Fish, and feeling dirty and slutty when I was done. To atone, the next day I ordered fish tacos, and ate the fish and cabbage and tomatoes but left the corn tortillas behind. I had had enough poison the day before. That experience made me realize something about the nature of exercise. The shorter, more intense workouts of CrossFit seemed to shut down my appetite, but longer, less intense efforts, like long rides or runs, left me famished. It was easy to undo the benefits of a two-hour bike ride in five minutes of gorging in the kitchen just after I had put my bike away. I could exercise less, albeit more intensely, and feel less hungry? Bring it.

Never, not once, during the two-month challenge did I ever feel tired or lethargic because of a lack of energy from a calorie deficit. In fact, I felt like I had more energy, and my mood was definitely better. Karianne urged us to look into periodic fasting, which was also part of the Paleo plan. But that smacked to me of food-weighing, and seemed like a recipe for crankiness, which I certainly didn't need any help with. I skipped it, even though she swore by it because the cavemen probably lived in feast-or-famine cycles of food supply.

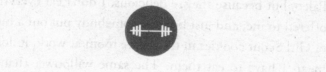

**C**rossFit Morristown's challenge experiment ended after two months. I lost a total of twenty pounds. Karianne urged us all to make this part of life. The word *diet* is derived from the Greek for "way of life," and the Paleo plan certainly seemed like a healthy way of life, one that was allowing me to climb ropes with greater ease and even to run a little bit faster. But to paraphrase Lincoln, the price of leanness is eternal vigilance. It took an enormous amount of concentration and planning to always eat this way. You have to plan ahead, all the time. You have to be conscious all the time. I know that's an excuse, and I know I'm lame for making it.

The instructors at my cert were right: it's nearly impossible to eat this way all the time, at least for me. It is exhausting. For me, it's better to allow yourself to cheat, and to know it's okay to do so once in a while, than to try to walk away forever from some of the things that give life its zest. There are zealots who would tell you that, yes, a piece of pie will kill you, actually. But I'm not one of them. I've decided to be pretty Paleo. I stick to the basic plan most of the time. I avoid sandwiches and pasta and rice and milk. I've added avocadoes to my diet, not just because they're Paleo, but because they're delicious. I don't eat everything offered to me, and just because somebody put out a bunch of Girl Scout cookies in the coffee room at work, it doesn't mean I have to eat them. The same willpower that gets me out of bed on a subzero morning to go do burpees has allowed me, most of the time, to walk past the offering of Halloween candy at the office reception desk. Not all the time, but more often than not.

I've decided that having cookies in my life once in a while means more to me than taking a minute off my time in the Grace WOD, in which you perform thirty clean-and-jerks as fast as you can. I've regained ten pounds, but my new pants still fit. I've made peace with the fact that I have traded some speed and agility for the ability to take advantage—to enjoy—some of the best things life has to offer me. Maybe that makes me a failure. Or maybe it makes me a well-rounded, happy guy who's more self-aware than he thought he was. I think it's the latter.

Of course, I have to remind myself of that deal I made with myself when I'm lying on the floor of the Annex, wondering why I'm not getting any faster at Grace. But like my breath, that knowledge eventually returns.

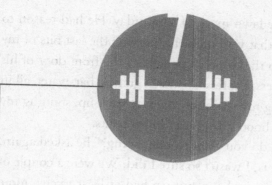

# The 20X

**D**o you want to keep going, Madden?"

The question came in like a distant AM radio station, broadcasting late at night. Filled with static, not entirely clear, alternately very loud and barely audible. It was the voice of Jim Rutan, the then-owner of CrossFit Honor, a box in Allentown, Pennsylvania. He was asking if I wanted to continue with the workout I had started a couple of hours ago, in the predawn murk of a Saturday. He had reason to ask: I was, at that very moment, heaving the last bits of my breakfast onto the wood chips next to the front door of his place of business. Espresso, banana, granola bar, water, all in a pile, burning my throat on the way back up, staining my black combat boots and green fatigue pants.

"Madden, do you want to keep going?" he asked again.

The truth is, I wasn't so sure I did. We were a couple of hours into this workout, but we had at least twelve more to go. I had signed up for the SEALFIT 20X Challenge, an all-day event I had come across online, taught by Commander Mark Divine, a former Navy SEAL, and a couple of his instructors, both also former SEALs. The come-on said that Divine and crew would show me that I was capable of twenty times more than I thought I was capable of, that the secret to being a high-achieving motherfucker was quieting, if not outright beating the shit out of, that little voice in the back of my head that kept telling me I was too tired or sore or fat or slow, that if I could just shut that off and let my body do its thing, I too could be okay. We would do this by completing three WODs in one fourteen-hour day, plus assorted other physical and mental activities. When it was over, I would be on my way to having an unbeatable mind. I would develop the mental toughness I needed, and that I knew I lacked. I was here for the mental toughness; I knew I could suffer through a day of this. I had spent the better part of the last few years beating down the voice that told me I was still slow and fat and didn't belong, that I should go back to my Matchbox cars. It was working. Now it was time to kill that voice once and for all. That's what I hoped to get out of the 20X.

Right this minute, though, that voice in my head was shouting through a megaphone aimed at my good ear, and it was very much coming through on digital FM. "You're not a Navy SEAL," it said. "You're a desk jockey. You're old. Just bail now and go home. You got a workout in. If you leave now, the other guys won't even miss you. Besides, you were dead fucking last in the mile run. You suck."

That's true. I do suck. But that doesn't mean I was ready to quit just then. Maybe in a little while. But not now. Who knew what else the day had in store. Besides, I had nothing left to puke.

"Let's go," I told Jim. "I got this."

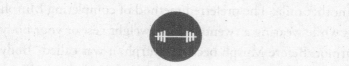

Spend any amount of time on Crossfit.com and it becomes very apparent that there's a strong connection between the program and the military. Not an official link, more like an affinity. The daily WOD posted on the site often includes a photo of an athlete in fatigues doing, for example, muscle-ups in some remote province of Afghanistan, or of sailors pumping improvised iron made of water jugs and rebar on the fantail of a ship at sea. CrossFit features a series of named workouts called "Hero WODs," standard workouts named for service members or first responders who have died in the line of duty. They tend to be the favorite workout of the people, almost all male, for whom they are named, and they can take on lives of their own.

"Murph" is a benchmark CrossFit workout named for Michael P. Murphy, a SEAL killed in Afghanistan in 2005 and posthumously awarded the Congressional Medal of Honor for valor in the operation described in Marcus Lutrell's book *Lone Survivor*. "Murph" goes like this: run one mile. Do 100 pull-ups, 200 push-ups, and 300 air squats. (You can partition the exercises and do 10 triads of 10 pull-ups, 20 push-ups, and 30 squats.) Then run another mile. The preferred method of completing Murph is while wearing a twenty-pound weight vest or your body armor. Before Murph became Murph, it was called "Body Armor," and became Murph after the SEAL's death. If you do it with the weight, it's called Heavy Murph. Either way, it offers a lot of suck to embrace, and it's at least part of the reason the CrossFit community has embraced Murph as a WOD to be done on Memorial Day to honor veterans. (To commemorate my fiftieth birthday in a few months, I will do Aquatic Murph, which replaces running the miles with swimming them, and substitutes a twenty-pound vest for six pounds in the pockets of my fatigues.)

It's not surprising that soldiers and firemen like Cross-Fit. It allows them to develop the intense, high-output, and brief bursts of power they need to do their jobs. It's far more likely that a fireman will have to run up a flight of stairs carrying a hose than it is that he'll need to run a 10K, or that a soldier will need to sprint across a field, drop to the ground, get up, and sprint again, the move at the base of a burpee.

I have to admit that the fact Navy SEALs were so into CrossFit was a big part of its appeal to me. SEALs are the ultimate cool guys, professional badasses, especially to someone who goes to meetings for a living. They're in great shape and get paid to stay that way. They jump out of airplanes and swim across open oceans, go scuba diving and ride around in minisubs. They pass insane physical and mental tests to get where they are, and have to be as tough inside as they are out. They blow up shit and hunt down bad guys and have every conceivable type of weapon known to a teenage boy. If they used CrossFit to maintain their impossibly high fitness standards, then it could be just the thing to vanquish once and for all the nagging voices in my head.

Of course, there's one massive, fundamental difference. Where the typical CrossFitter will do a daily WOD and then spend the rest of the day behind a desk or chasing around after kids, the SEALs' lives are one giant WOD, an endless series of burpees, runs, swims, and pull-ups, combined with a lack of sleep and hot food. Granted, they are superb specimens, mostly young men with energy to burn. But I was in pretty good shape, and I had a lifetime of training and muscle memory. If I could find a group offering a SEAL experience, I thought, maybe I could finally prove, once and for all, that I was good enough. It wasn't like the world was looking at me—friends, colleagues, and family—and saying all this. It all was within me, that voice inside my head from long ago, one I should have quieted by now. I was fucking sick of it. I was pushing it off with each WOD I completed. If I could get through the 20X, chances are it would be gone for good. Or so I hoped.

The day had started innocently enough. It was foggy and dark in Allentown, Pennsylvania, with cold rain in the forecast and standing puddles of water on both the pavement and the grass around the gym, tucked away in an industrial park. Fourteen people had gathered at the box, dressed in the required fatigues, boots, and white T-shirts with our names scrawled in Magic Marker across the chest and back. Be ready to go at 6 a.m., the "warning orders" email had told us, so at 5:45 a.m. we stood in loose circles, checking each other out, idly stretching. The average age of the participants was about twenty-eight. Most were barrel-chested and thick-armed. A single woman stood out, her hair pulled into a tight double braid. At forty-nine, I wasn't the oldest person; that honor belonged to a guy who loudly let us know he was both a doctor and a captain in the National Guard. Clearly, I thought, he was angling to be the guy everybody would fall in behind and follow for the rest of the day. While I wasn't looking to lead, I wasn't about to blindly follow someone I didn't know, someone whose primary qualification so far seemed to be a big mouth. I was more likely to follow someone who over the course of the day would prove with his actions that he or she knew what he or she was doing. I gathered from snatches of overheard conversation that at least some of the younger guys, including a cadet from the U.S. Naval Academy, hoped to become SEALs.

This is the point where I had my usual pre-event "What the fuck am I doing here?" moment. Whether it's looking over a body of water I was about to swim across or at a distant mountain peak I was about to climb, an empty office at a start-up or at a bride walking down the aisle toward me, the thought that I have well and truly finally gotten myself in over my head has been a constant in my life. It was certainly the case this morning, as I looked at the far fitter people around me, at the pull-up bars and weights and tires and massive logs and sandbags and rucksacks that I knew we would be impaling ourselves on here today. It's a shitty way to start a day. This will be the last time I ever ask myself this question, I thought. When today is over, I'll know exactly why I'm here. I came for answers.

At 5:59 the big-mouth doctor had us come to attention in neat military rows, anticipating the prompt arrival of our instructors. This is why they draft young guys, I thought. Old dogs don't like being told what to do.

We stood like that, quietly, for five minutes. Ten. Fifteen. Twenty. Doc told us to stand at ease, still military style. More time passed. All part of the head games, I thought. Keep us waiting. Make us get all squirrelly, thinking, dreading. Well, it worked. I was thinking, and I was dreading. Use this time to get your shit together, one side of my brain thought. Use this time to panic and think of excuses for why you should bail and go to a Starbucks, came the reply from the other. All the while, my stomach gurgled. Against my better judgment, and all my experience, I had drunk two espressos at 4 a.m. before I left home, figuring everything would be digested by the time we got to the rough stuff.

Then, about 6:45 or so, the door opened and two guys, both very fit looking, one looking to be just a little bit older than the other, calmly and quietly entered the box. They wore standard-issue cool outdoor guy apparel. The older one was in a puffy down jacket, sweatpants, and army boots, and had sunglasses perched atop his head despite the predawn darkness; the younger had on a black watch cap and a fleece jacket, and wore shorts and running shoes despite the chill. The older one was pretty big. The other was surprisingly short. They immediately circled us slowly, telling us how out of shape and undedicated we were. I didn't need to pay four hundred dollars to learn that, I thought. Then they had us drop into a push-up position and stay there.

That's when Mark Divine walked through the door. I don't think it's possible for me to describe Divine without sounding like I have a boy crush. Tall, ramrod straight, impressively built, and oddly ageless, Divine moved silently and with complete control. If he said anything at that point, I don't remember what it was. I just recall being struck by his command presence. Forget the loud-mouth doctor; this was a guy I'd follow anywhere. This was a guy who had seen shit. Who knew shit. Good, I thought. Here was the sensei I had come to learn from.

Divine walked around our group and explained how the day would go. We'd work out, a lot. We'd get some instruction on keeping our focus and remaining strong, both physically and mentally. There wouldn't be a ton of yelling, he said, because we were all adults, and they had plenty of ways to get our attention without yelling. They had some surprises for us, and we had some surprises for ourselves. If we paid attention, and gave ourselves over fully to the process, we'd get what we came for.

They then proceeded to yell at us. A lot. Stand here. Do this. Do the push-ups as a group. As a group, goddammit. Every time someone screwed up because he or she wasn't listening, we did push-ups.

We did a lot of push-ups. There was more yelling. Keep your head up so you can look around. Keep your ass down. Feet together. Hands in.

But because I knew it was coming, and because I wasn't tired, I didn't care about the yelling, and I certainly didn't take it personally when the instructors yelled at me or criticized me. All part of the process, I thought. Plus, when it's all over later today, I get to go home and sleep in my own bed. It's not like I'm really in the navy, or a SEAL.

Before signing me up for the 20X, someone at SEAL-FIT headquarters had emailed me to be sure I could pass the minimum fitness standards: run a mile in army boots and long pants on a road in less than ten minutes; do at least forty each of push-ups, sit-ups, and air squats in two minutes or less. So one Sunday about a month before the camp, I went out to the garage and knocked them all out. No problem.

Oh, one other thing: men should be able to do eight dead-hang pull-ups. Problem. Just like at last summer's Warrior Challenge, I still sucked at pull-ups. I worked on them, using bands of varying strengths to provide a boost, buying a contraption made of surgical tubing to help, pulling myself up whenever I walked by a suitable bar, reading about tricks to use to incorporate other muscles into the lift. My dead hangs had, in fact, improved, from a maximum of three to a maximum of six. But six ain't eight. The simple fact was that until I could figure out a way to use my quads and my ass to do pull-ups, a long shot, or until I lost another twenty pounds, a longer shot, I was going to be pull-up challenged.

So I told the people at SEALFIT that the dead hangs could be a problem, the other stuff was fine, and they said okay, come on down anyway. I kept doing CrossFit to prepare for the camp, and everything seemed fine.

Until our instructors told us it was time to demonstrate our proficiency at the fitness standards. Both instructors started yelling about how it pays to be a winner and that standards are just that, bare minimums, and did we want to live a life of bare minimums? Didn't we want to excel, not just at this but at every thing we did? In fact, a life devoid of dead-hang pull-ups was fine with me, but if today I was supposed to do as many as I could, then I'd do as many as I could. Hell, one of the other guys did seventeen.

Once again, I did three.

The shorter instructor came over to me. "What's the problem"—and here he looked straight at my chest to read my name—"Madden?"

Here I was tempted to say, Fuck off, there is no problem. But images of a day spent on this guy's wrong side, of a day of punitive push-ups, flashed through my head, so I thought better of that, and said, "I did three pull-ups, coach." (There was no way was I calling anybody sir.)

"That's it?" His eyebrows arched above the rims of his horn-rimmed glasses, the ones that made me think of

David Byrne in the video for "Once in a Lifetime." I was scared. It was the first and only time David Byrne has ever scared anybody.

"Yes, sir," I stammered.

"You know you were supposed to be able to do eight? You had all this time to prepare and you come here not ready? What else can't you do, Madden? Why are you even here?"

This I was ready for. This I had thought about. The simple, glib answer was that I wanted to be mentally tougher and was here to learn the secrets of America's steely warrior class. But the real answers were far more complex. There were the voices that needed to be quelled. And I wanted to be able to deal with a bunch of bosses—due to the structure of the joint venture I ran, I had four of them—who were, at this particular point in the development of my website, skull-fucking me with random emails, criticisms, complaints, and general expressions of unhappiness with me and my performance. If they were unhappy with me, they might fire me. If they fired me, I wouldn't be able to provide for my family, for my children. So if I were mentally tougher, I'd be able to get those guys off my back, or at the very least pay less attention to them. I'd keep my job and the Madden kids would be able to eat meat a couple of times a week and go to the college of their choices. At least that's how me and my squirrel brain saw it.

"I'm here to be a better father," I said.

It was clear from the look on his face that it was not the answer he was expecting. Nor was it really the answer I was expecting. But all the hours of going to bed before the kids and of being too tired to really and truly engage them the way I had hoped I would as a father, of wanting desperately to not fuck up and be the dad who told them I wasn't going to drive them to a bike race and what made them think they could even do a bike race anyhow, distilled the complexities of my thoughts to a seven-word answer. He paused, smirked. "Go do the push-ups," he said.

I passed the push-ups test, pumping out 58, unbroken, in two minutes. Squats? I scoff at squats. I did 75 squats so picture perfect you could have charged people cash money to see them. The sit-ups? A mere 35. But I had a reason. An excuse, really, but the instructors had told us this was an excuse-free zone, excuses being like assholes, blah blah blah: they had us do the type of sit-up in which a partner holds your feet, which you place flat on the ground while your hands go behind your head. I trained for CrossFit sit-ups, in which you place a pad called an AbMat at the small of your back, put the soles of your feet together, and reach your hands way out behind your head when you go back and in front of your feet when you go forward.

The big instructor wrote everyone's totals on a whiteboard. Some of the guys had crushed the standards, with upwards of two hundred reps. I was DFL: dead fucking last. Even the big mouth had beaten me. "Remember these numbers," the instructor said. "It's always really interesting to see who can bring it now, and who can bring it eight hours from now." I took solace in that thought. I'm a total second-half guy.

Then we ran the mile. I used to love running. I was a decent 400-meter guy in high school. I've completed two marathons and countless shorter road races. But I have come to hate running with a passion. Part of it has to do with the fact that every time I run, with every step I remember the feeling of running away from all those kids to score the touchdown that night in Norwood. Now I'm not running away from anybody. I used to like this. And now it sucks. I'm slow, watching those Hatfields again.

It sure sucked at the 20X. As the others roared off, I fought to maintain contact with the back of the group. Then I fought to maintain sight of them. This was bad. By the time I had reached the turnaround at the halfway point, the espresso that I thought would be out of my system by now suddenly seemed very, very present as it bubbled in the back of my throat.

I could hear, barely, the sound of someone running up behind me. "Looking good, Madden." It was Divine. "Breathe, nice and easy. Lean forward, almost like you're falling forward. Land on the balls of your feet, not flat-footed. You got this." It was reassuring to have Divine there, a half step ahead of me, urging me on. It was also embarrassing. Here I was, once again, the fat kid who couldn't keep up, who needed help. I wasn't sure what had happened between the day I tested myself and this, but I felt the sudden urge to stop. I slowed even more. "Do *not* stop," Divine warned. He hadn't raised his voice one bit, but the emphasis was more than enough to keep me moving, even as bile crept up my throat. "Come on. Just to that post up there." Then "Just to that driveway. You got this, Madden. You got this."

"You don't have this. Just stop," said one voice in my head.

"Don't stop," said a slightly louder one.

Step after agonizing step I listened to the louder one. I didn't want to embarrass myself further in front of the ultimate Cool Guy. Thoughts of regret for that breakfast filled my brain, then the breakfast itself filled my throat. But I kept running.

Finally, we reached the door of the box. Divine walked silently inside, where I could see the others gathered, already recovered, sipping from water bottles. That's when I started barfing, and when Rutan asked if I wanted to continue. He was concerned. I wasn't.

I was used to this, and I knew I'd feel better afterward. And as disgusting and disconcerting as it may have been to a stranger, and as off-putting, to me it was just another day at this particular office.

So, yeah. "I'm okay. I got this."

The rest of the morning unfolded in a series of exercises

and lectures, all designed to reinforce the main tenet of SEALFIT: You can do more than you think you can, and you can do way more than you think you can if you work as a team, with each individual giving his or her maximum effort while playing to your individual strengths, as long as the team has a plan going into the task. Rather than seeing this whole thing as a competition between individuals, we should, Divine said, figure out a way to use each other's strengths while minimizing our weaknesses. We read aloud the SEAL creed, and we read "Invictus," the hoary old staple of high school yearbooks that, in this setting, seemed less like a source of inspirational quotes and more of a mission statement: "I am the master of my fate. I am the captain of my soul." Whether I succeeded or failed was entirely up to me. No voice in my head could tell me what to do or hold me back if I didn't want it to. Run or quit, the choice was mine. With each successive exercise, and each successive lecture, the SEALFIT guys were reinforcing the message that teams succeeded because of individual effort, and individuals succeeded because the team succeeded. But true success only came when every single person on the team worked as hard and as smart as they could—they put out—because they knew their teammates were doing the same. Strong members would help weaker members, because they knew that sooner or later the roles would be reversed somehow.

Divine told us that SEALs need to be able to do three things at the same time, and do them well: shoot their weapons effectively, move, and communicate with other team members. We didn't have weapons, but we did move a lot, and communication—not often a strong point among men, and certainly not in what, despite all their exhortations to teamwork, remained a competitive environment—wasn't a strong point.

The best example of this came midmorning. A Cross-Fit gym is a repository of a staggering amount of stuff: pairs of dumbbells of all weights and sizes, medicine balls, AbMats, jump ropes, barbells, weight plates, yoga mats, stretching bands, giant tires, sledgehammers, sandbags, racks to put all this stuff on. Divine divided us up into two teams and told us to move all the stuff at one end of the gym to the other as fast as we could, and to keep an inventory of everything we moved.

Sounds easy, but it's not. The first impulse of almost everyone on the team was to grab a piece of the gear and run it to the other end of the gym. But wait: Would it be faster to make a bucket chain? Who was keeping track of all this stuff? Could we just leave the weights on the racks and roll them down, making one very sweaty trip instead of ten less sweaty trips? The trick, Divine said: before you do anything, make a plan and designate responsibilities, and work together. Somehow, I ended up as the scribe, keeping track of everything and noting counts on a whiteboard, playing to my strengths while minimizing the effect of my weaknesses on the team.

The same lessons were reinforced when each team was assigned a giant log. Hurricane Sandy had recently blown through the area and had decimated the local forests, so Rutan had found two beautiful logs, each weighing about five hundred pounds. They had been shaved of their bark and sanded smooth. One was christened Inspiration, the other Perspiration. Each team had to work together to lift the log from the ground to right shoulder height, then overhead, then to the left shoulder, then down, then back over the top. We also sat on the ground, held the log at chest level, and did sit-ups as a group. If we didn't work as one, if we didn't communicate, we didn't complete the lift. It took a while, but we eventually got the hang of it and started to feel like a team. As proof, Divine had us hold the log up on one end and support it as a unit while one of our teammates climbed the log and sat on top. There was no way I thought this would be possible. But it was. There was our guy, on top of Old Inspiration, laughing down at us. I was starting to get the sense that we really were all capable of more than we thought.

Lunch was put out for us, and I chose wisely, a few carrots, an energy bar, half a turkey sandwich, and about a gallon of water. We ate in hurried bites and were told to change from our sweaty clothes into warmer, drier clothes: we were headed outside.

"The good news," said the older instructor, who we now knew was named Bruce, "is that it's one p.m. You've made it this far. The bad news is that it's only one p.m."

At that point, we donned cheap little rucksacks filled with 10 percent of our body weight in sand. We were then handed PVC pipes filled with another fourteen pounds of sand. "This is how much your weapon would weigh were you to be issued one in Afghanistan," he said. We headed out the door, in a line behind Bruce, and we started to walk. Fast. Then we started to run. Bruce led us along the side of the road in the industrial park. Then down into a drainage ditch. Around trees. Back to the road. Across the road. Up and down. The most disconcerting thing was having no idea of where we were going, or how long this was going to last. It just . . . it just was. This was what I was doing today. As much as it sucked to try to keep up with Bruce, who moved effortlessly, I was okay with it. There was a lot of yelling about staying together and working as a unit, about taking a turn carrying the huge rope we had brought. It was raining. It sucked. But so what? I was giving in to it and embracing the suck.

Eventually, we got to a park where we took turns hiding and hunting each other down. Basically, you had to burrow under the wet leaves and lie there until somebody stumbled over you. The basic lesson: don't think that if you cover yourself with wet leaves you'll be hidden from view. Work together. Have someone else cover you so you're well and truly hidden. Be a team.

Lying under the wet leaves was surprisingly warm, though, and gave me a half hour or so to relax and recover, and to think. This isn't so bad. I can get through the rest of this. I can take anything for a few more hours, right? I wish I had a Snickers bar right now. Fuck that Paleo shit. I wonder what Anne and the kids are doing. How are all my friends at home? And this one, from near the stem of my brain: There's no way the Hatfields could do this. No way. This was all me.

Then it was on to a tug-of-war, and a team exercise to get everyone up into a massive tree using the rope. The highlight of this exercise was when one of the two South African guys in the group fell from about fifteen feet up, hit the ground with an impressive sigh as the air left his lungs, and got back up to eventually rejoin the group. Talk about never quitting a workout. Hard-fucking-core.

I started to fade on the run back to the box. A younger, much fitter teammate named Paul—first name? last name? I still don't know—kept his hand on my back and pushed me the whole way. It was a huge boost. The contact, the support, the energy, the acknowledgment that I wasn't doing as well as the rest but was still putting out. This was being a good teammate, a good guy. This was looking out for people.

Finally, finally, we returned to the box and changed again, this time into shorts and T-shirts, then gathered around the whiteboard, which this time featured a photograph of a sailor in dress uniform, and a workout, whom we all recognized as Murph. This, we were told, was the central part of the 20X experience, because Murph epitomized what being a good teammate was all about. And our three instructors had all known Murph.

Instructor Brad read aloud the citation that accompanied Murph's Medal of Honor as we stood around, tired and sore, knowing what was coming: a mile run, 100 pull-ups, 200 push-ups, 300 squats, and another mile run. All on top of the hours that had gone before. The citation wasn't exactly the St. Crispin's Day Speech, but it had the same effect on us. It described how Murph, as part of a four-man team sent to a mountain village to capture a local Taliban leader, had exposed himself to enemy fire in order to catch a clear radio signal back to headquarters to request additional support when they had lost the element of surprise. "Murph knew that by doing that he could get hit, but he did it anyway," Brad said, before saying, "and yeah, he got hit, and he died."

Divine spoke up. "We take this workout very, very seriously," he said. "It's a way for us, for you, to honor Murph's sacrifice. All that we ask of you here is everything that you have. Just like Murph."

We donned our sand-filled rucks and started. This mile felt different from the sufferfest of the morning, though. I wasn't any faster, but I wasn't in uncharted territory. I had done Murph before, and knew I had about seventy minutes of putting out ahead of me. So I ran. I ran and I didn't stop. I wasn't the last guy back into the box. The mile took just more than ten minutes.

I partitioned the workout, as most people do, into ten sets: 10 pull-ups, 20 push-ups, 30 squats. The pull-ups were agony, and within a few sets, I was really struggling. Instructor Brad, the guy with the David Byrne glasses, was back at my side. Fuck, I thought. Here it comes. More shit.

"Come on, Madden, you got this," he said, leaning in, his voice devoid of the sharp edges that had defined it before. "You can do it. Use this box. Step up and grab the bar."

Something had turned, in both me and the instructors. I had tried all day, applied myself, put out, didn't complain. I knew I was no standout—in fact, I was probably one of the weakest guys here—but I tried as hard as I could. And that was what they wanted. It's what I wanted from myself. I don't know this for a fact, but my sense was that rather than beat us down, now that they saw that we were serious, they were building us up. I paused and looked around the room. It seemed to be happening everywhere.

"Here, use this band," Brad said, slipping a giant rubber band—like the ones I used at the Annex—over the bar, which became a giant slingshot to help me get my chin up and over. Total cheating. To make up for this, I did hand-release push-ups. Basically, when you lower yourself to the ground, you lift your hands up. There's no way to cheat. When Bruce and Brad told me I was making it harder on myself, I said it was to make up for the boost on the pull-ups. They didn't say anything.

I had made it a goal to do each group of thirty squats unbroken: not stopping once I had started a set. The squats felt easy. Was I warmed up? Was I channeling Murph? I don't know, but I knew I wasn't DFL this time. The squats were unbroken. When I finished the second mile, I had completed Murph heavy in 1:06. Some twenty minutes behind the fastest guys, but five minutes faster than I ever had before.

It was dark by the time they rolled up the garage door at the back of the gym and told us to assemble at the edge of the parking lot, above a rock-strewn gully. I didn't know what time it was, but to judge by the darkness, I figured we had maybe an hour to go. Maybe two at the most. Piece of cake. Chip away. Something big and bad had to be coming. But, I told myself again, I got this.

Divine had us stand at attention while he explained that we were all to go down into the gully to find a rock that represents our will to live. We were told to bring our chosen rock back up to the parking lot.

So we stumbled down over the rocks, which ranged in size from pieces of gravel to boulders. I was looking for the biggest fucking rock I could find. Because by now I know that I'm not going to quit, whatever it is, and I'm not going to be broken and that if things get bad, I can lean on the other guys.

I found one, a monster, but whether it was the size of the rock or the sum total of the day's exertions, I couldn't get it up the slope. Weird. Back at CrossFit, I can throw around a 125-pound sack of sand. I stared at the rock, as if my gaze would make it levitate. It didn't.

"Come on, Madden," says Instructor Brad from above.

"I'm moving this rock that represents my will to survive," I say. Under his breath, in a conspiratorial hush, he tells me, "Find a smaller one, you asshole. You have to carry it for a mile."

So that's the grand finale.

I found a smaller one, about seventy-five pounds, I guess. My will to live remained huge, but more portable. Then the order came: We are to pick up the rock and start walking. If one of us drops his or her rock, we all start over. Don't drop the fucking rock.

No problem. What's a mile?

But first, we took turns immersing ourselves, one at a time, head and all, in a barrel of ice-cold water. We helped each other climb up and in, duck under, and breathe out until bubbles show. Helping each other kept our minds off the shivering. Instructor Bruce stood behind the barrel to make sure we were all the way under, and under for a good long time.

Why? Because why not? What's one more thing? Plus, of all the stuff we did that day, being under the water, and cold, and wet, played to my strengths. I noticed I wasn't shivering as much as the skinny guys. All that fat finally coming in handy. When some of the shivering got out of control for some of the guys, the instructors had us stand

138

in a huddle, the stomachs and chests of the bigger guys braced against the backs of the smaller ones. The heat transferred as if conducted by wire. I was at the very back, my girth finally helping my teammates. I noticed my chest was pressing against Paul's back. His shivering stopped.

"You're better off together than you are alone!" one of the instructors yelled. "Remember that."

We carried the rocks in laps around the building. We stayed together, urging each other on. There was a lot of groaning, and screaming, and shifting of the rock from shoulder to shoulder and from waist to back as we all sought a comfortable place to rest our burdens. We stumbled through the darkness, the glare of the sodium lights bathing us in pink. Wet, chafing, suddenly no longer cold. Sweating again.

We finished. And we lined up.

"You can put the rocks down," Divine said. He told us to take a knee next to our rocks. Divine walked slowly to the end of the line opposite me and said, "I want you all to think of an answer to this question: what's the most important thing you've learned in the past year?"

I thanked God I was at the other end of the line. I knew I should be listening to my teammates, learning from their answers, and one small part of my brain did, hearing them talk about never stopping, never quitting, but I couldn't think of anything to say but at least now I'll have some time to think as he works his way down the line. What's my answer? What was the most important thing I learned in the last year? Was it something from the last fourteen hours? The last twelve months? About hard work and fighting and being smart and not quitting and staying true to your word, to promises made, even if they were unsaid? To myself, to my family? My mind raced, but my mental tires spun in the mud of my fatigue. I have no answer, I think.

"Madden?" Divine is in front of me. "What's the most important thing you learned this year?"

I wish I could say it was a carefully, consciously constructed thought. I wish I could say my brain played, in a flash, a two-hour movie of my kids, my wife, my family, my coworkers, my brothers and sisters and anybody who ever helped me and whom I ever helped. All the people I love, and who love me. I wish I could say my fine, educated mind delivered the thought. But the truth is, I just blurted it out.

"Love is the answer, sir."

Divine scares me, staring at me through the murk of a February night. He must think I'm putting him on or being a wise guy. Who talks to a Navy SEAL about love? He's gonna make me take another lap with the rock. And you know what? That's okay. At this point, I know I can do it. I can take anything he wants to dish out. I'd rather not, but I can if I have to. I'm fine with it. Because at this point, I know my answer is right. Love is the answer. If I didn't love my family, why would I have done this? And if I didn't love myself, how could I have done this.

He's still looking at me. "Outstanding, Madden. Outstanding."

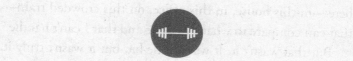

I was utterly depleted by the 20X. I drove the ninety miles home, surprisingly alert after what I had been through, while I cataloged the different places and ways I was sore. When I got home, I pounded a shot of good tequila and chased it with a beer and a handful of ibuprofen to quell the swelling I knew was coming. I had a fitful night's sleep; anytime I rolled over, my body screamed at the effort and soreness and woke me from the shallow trough of slumber I had managed to crawl in to. It took almost a week for my body to recover sufficiently to start WODing again.

But if I was utterly depleted, I was also utterly at peace, the peace that passes all understanding. For a week after the 20X, I felt as if I were floating, as if I had attained some sort of neutral buoyancy in the river of my life that was allowing me to feel, for the first and only time, that I really was okay, and that I could accept things and people, particularly myself, as they were. I really was capable of anything. I could deal with the bosses. College? We'll get you through, kids. Don't worry. Nothing bothered me. I laughed easily. I slept like a rock. An easy assessment would have been something like, "I've been through the shit, man, and there's nothing here—in this house, in this office, on this crowded train—that can compare to what I've done and that I can't handle."

But that wasn't it. It was a little bit, but it wasn't truly it. Looking back now, with the clarity of retrospect, I can see what the source of the peace was. After almost fifty years of trying to figure out what the point of all this was, I had stumbled across an answer that was right in front of me the whole time, or had it pulled out of me: love really is the answer.

There was another benefit. One morning at the Annex about ten days after the 20X, we were practicing a move called a Turkish get-up. Basically, you hold a weight up over your head with a single straight arm. You then lower yourself to the ground, lying flat out with the weight extended in the air above your head. Then you get back up. The heavier or more awkward the weight, the harder it is to get up. This morning I decided to try the weight with a long 45-pound Olympic bar rather than the less awkward and more conventional kettle bell. I had never been able to do a Turkish get-up with a bar. But this morning I resolved to do five with each arm. My entire body said no with each rep. It said to put the bar down and get a kettle bell.

But my mind said yes. And my mind won.

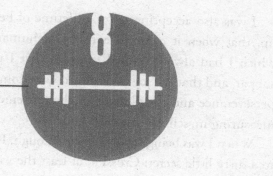

# Nine Days in May

I had done the 20X to make myself mentally tougher. I was doing CrossFit to see what I was really made of. But what I was learning was that I was made of perfectly ordinary muscles and bones, but that it was my spirit, my desire to be a better husband and a better father, a better friend, a better teammate and coworker, that was pushing me.

I was also accepting, after a lifetime of beating myself up, that when it came to a realm of human activity in which I had always wanted to excel, that I was perfectly subpar, and that the joy and reward were coming from the perseverance and the pleasure of the movement, not from measuring myself against everybody else

When I was being totally honest, though, I had to admit to a dirty little secret: CrossFit, at least the way I practiced it, was starting to wear me down. The 5:30 a.m. starts were killing me again, and being in bed by 9:30 on weekdays and falling asleep on the couch by ten on weekends wasn't winning me any points with my family. If I were doing my four or five workouts a week at noon, or even after work, it might be a different story, and it seemed to be for Anne, who went at 8:45 a.m., after the kids went to school. But while she was thriving, I was stalled. I had hit some plateaus. I wasn't getting any faster running, my one-rep maxes on most weights weren't going any higher, double unders were intermittent, and my muscle-ups were stalled at the pull-up phase.

Still, I felt strong, and in the best shape of my life. I could throw around weights I could never dream of lifting before, I could go off and do pretty much any physical activity I wanted to, and I looked better than I ever had. And I felt good. Plus, basic little fitness tests told the story. I could walk up stairs two at a time with no effort. I could stand up from a chair without touching the arms, and my general balance was as good as it had ever been.

One of the basic goals of CrossFit is to get you ready for whatever life throws at you. I learned the hard way when I worked at *Bicycling* that relying on any single exercise movement can get you in very good shape—for that single exercise movement—but that if you want to be an all-arounder, you need to mix it up. CrossFit does that in spades, through its credo of constantly varying the motions and exercises we do. But after all the time in the box, I wanted to feel the sun on my back, and to test myself in a variety of ways I can't do when always in a gym. It was time to take it outside, and to see what was under the hood. I wanted to play with my fitness, and with my friends and family.

I wasn't the only one at the Annex who was feeling that way. Mickey had organized a team to compete on May 18 in the Civilian Military Challenge (CMC), a race that consisted of a seven-minute WOD followed immediately by a five-mile cross-country run strewn with natural and man-made obstacles laid out on a ski slope in the Poconos. By coincidence, my family and I had entered an open-water swim to be held on our annual trip to St. John the following weekend. And somewhere in there, the Annex would be completing a Murph. If I took part in all the fun, I would be beating the shit out of myself over just nine days. We don't run that much during our winter programming at the Annex, and I hadn't been swimming much, at all. But I was always beating the shit out of myself. Now was the time to test the fitness, and to test whether I really had quelled the bad voice in my head.

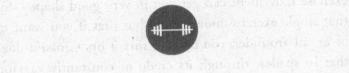

Camelback Mountain is a small ski area in the Pocono Mountains of eastern Pennsylvania. Once a region known for producing the coal that fueled the furnaces of nearby Bethlehem Steel, the forge that produced the framework of the Brooklyn Bridge, the Empire State Building, and a fleet of battleships, the Poconos now are a ticky-tacky tourist mecca filled with designer outlet malls, low-stakes casinos, fudge stands, and taxidermy shops that cater to the hunters who flow in there every deer season. None of this detracts, however, from the harsh steepness of the thousand-foot hills (*mountain* being a relative term here) or the seemingly endless piles and fields of rocks strewn across them. This is where we'd be racing. In addition to 166 acres of skiable terrain, Camelback, in a nod to increasing the length of its season, had built a water park, whose wave tanks, flumes, and feeder ponds would serve as some of the obstacles in the race. That boded well for me; water was my great equalizer.

Team Annex consisted of two men: me and Mickey,

and six women. And the women were ready to kick some ass.

The core group of women who work out at the Annex are the 35–50-year-old suburban mom equivalents of the Type A guys who make up the 5:30 WOD. Hypereducated executives turned stay-at-home moms, they are fire breathers in yoga pants and sports bras, former college athletes who compete at everything they do—CrossFit, running a school fund-raiser, managing the funds of the town Cub Scout troop—with a ferocity that would put Michael Jordan to shame. They may not lift the same amount of weights as the guys, but they can run as fast if not faster than most of them, and pump out pull-ups, double unders, box jumps, and burpees like marines. They are badass, all business at the box, and if they weren't home raising their broods, they would be ruling the world.

I am married to one of them. Anne and I met on a blind date, set up by friends who knew we were both into, in Dan's words, "all that running and swimming shit." Anne had taken up running in high school and had been on the track and cross-country teams at Williams College, where she learned how to shake off the previous night's party by running ten miles up and down the trails in the Berkshire Mountains. Working out was a regular part of her life before I met her, and it was part of what drew us together. We got engaged on a hiking trip to Washington State. We honeymooned with a sea kayaking trip to Hawaii, after we had given each other new road bikes as wedding presents.

We would always make time to work out, even after we had three kids in two years. We made it a point to exercise with the kids, even getting a triple baby jogger to push Luke, Catherine, and Christine on runs through Chatham. We'd take turns pushing, trading off a backpack filled with diapers, formula, and blankets, all in the name of getting out of the house and staying in some sort of shape. We must have looked absurd.

That Anne was a better athlete than me never bothered me too much. I was part of a generation of boys who were starting to get the message that if it was okay for girls to be smarter than us in school or have better positions in the student council, then it only followed that a girl could run you into the ground, too. Anne could run me into the ground, do more sit-ups, and ride away from me on a bike. I could swim better than she could, but that was just because I had been swimming longer.

But now, as she stood with them in a loose circle at the parking lot of Camelback's base lodge, she scared me. They all scared me. We were there as Team Annex, and I knew there was no way I was going to be able to keep up with them. Any of them. I would be the weak link. I would be the drift anchor. I would be the one they stood waiting for, impatiently checking their watches as precious seconds ticked by, seconds that defined how you compared to the other people who were here, seconds that defined who you were and where you stood in the world. I would be pissing them off. And I didn't want to do that. You don't want to piss off the suburban she-wolves.

"Hey, guys," I said, as we contorted our legs into stretches, already planning my out as I surveyed the rest of the field, which was uniformly younger, fitter, and more tattooed than Team Annex. "I was thinking that maybe we should do this not so much like a team where we all run together but more like a cross-country meet where everyone just goes for it and our individual points count at the end, you know?"

"No, we're all here together, we can do it together," Muffie said, hopping from one foot to the next. *Muffie, mother of five, former college lacrosse player, former network sales executive, is a machine.* I didn't know how she'd do on the water obstacles we'd face, or on the walls we'd have to scale, but when it came to running and just about anything else, I knew she'd eat me alive. "It will be fine." Here comes the ass-kicking. Mark Divine and his band of former SEALs could put a hurt on me that I knew I could endure. But I knew I'd never see any of those people again. I saw some of these women—say, for example, my wife— every day.

The first challenge we faced was the CMC Pit. It was a seven-minute WOD in which we were to do as many reps as possible of seven kettle bell swings, seven burpee box jumps, and seven strict presses. We had practiced this WOD a few times at the Annex, programming it in to the daily WOD so people would know what to expect. Here at the Pit, each athlete had his own station and judge, who was there to offer encouragement but mainly to make sure we did each and every rep strictly by the rules. They could "no-count" us if one of our feet didn't go over the top of the box on the box jump, or if our ears didn't show in front of our arms on the kettle bell swings. There were some sixty workstations in the Pit, overseen by a DJ connected to an extremely large sound system that pumped out the speed-metal-meets-rap music that formed CrossFit's sound track.

Athletes entered the Pit, a rectangle defined by crowd-control barriers in the ski area parking lot, in groups of sixty, and ran to a vacant workstation. Team Annex entered as one. But I wanted to be far back from the barriers, because I didn't want any spectators gawking at me. I didn't want the distraction. My plan was to start slowly, easily, build into the workout, and make sure I didn't blow up. As I jogged toward a nondescript station, head down, I felt a tap on my shoulder. "Hey 20X!" a voice called. It was familiar, but I couldn't place it beyond knowing it had something to do with both pain and encouragement. Strange. I stopped and looked, and there was the muscular fireplug who had put his hand on my back and willed me through the last stages of the ruck at the SEALFIT 20X with his gentle "You got this, Madden." It was Paul. And he was a judge. My judge.

We hugged like we were brothers, which was weird. I still didn't know if Paul was this guy's last name or first name. All I knew is that he had it stenciled on his T-shirt at the 20X, front and back, the way I had Madden stenciled on mine. But we hugged and backslapped and yelled as if we had been through a hell together, a hell nobody else but those who had endured it could understand. Up until that point, I had considered the 20X a very hard one-day event, one that taught me a lot. But the pure elation and surprise I felt at seeing this guy who had helped me so much, who had given of himself so that we could finish as a team, who had helped me arrive at the answer, knocked me back on my heels. Any trace of doubt I had felt, or fear of getting my ass kicked, evaporated as soon as Paul told me, "Madden, you have so got this."

I settled in with my hands on the kettle bell, my ass in a low squat, weight on my heels. Paul asked how many reps I thought I could get in seven minutes, and I told him my best efforts so far had yielded ninety or so. "You look fit and you're psyched, right?" he shouted over the amplified din. I assured him I was. "Get ready to break one hundred," he said.

"Three, two, one, GO!"

I still don't know the primary source of the roaring in my ears. Was it Paul, screaming encouragement? The music, played at a stadiumlike decibel level? The sound of my own heartbeat? I pumped out the seven kettle bell swings and immediately dropped to the ground to begin the burpees. Unlike a regular burpee, in which you just jump up and clap your hands over your head, the Pit version called for us to jump up onto a twenty-inch box, stand up straight, then jump back down and do it again. I did, as Paul screamed and the announcer roared about how well Team Annex was doing. I finished the burpees, grabbed the barbell, cleaned it into the high rack, and pumped out seven push-presses. After one round, it was clear: the burpees would kill me. I needed to get through the kettle bell swings and the presses as steadily as possible and focus on the burpees. Paul sensed it, too, and ratcheted up his encouragement when I did the burpees, but delivered a smooth, modulated stream of "Yes, yes, yes" while I did the others. Two rounds. Three rounds done and 3:30 to go. Could I possibly be headed to 120 reps? Oh my God. I felt so good. I was strong, and Paul knew it. Everyone knew it. I was flying.

Until I wasn't. At once, I felt as if a bomb of lactic acid had gone off deep inside me, and was sending its muscle-stopping shock waves out through my trunk, my limbs, my hands and feet, my scalp. The trick now was to beat the waves and get as many reps in as I could. I bent over to grab the kettle bell and blew out, three steady breaths. "Don't stop! Don't stop!" Paul screamed. I stood up "Don't let go! Get reps! Go!" Paul was crazed. He wanted me to break one hundred more than I did, and he didn't care that I was gassed. I didn't care if I broke one hundred, but Paul seemed to care very much for me, and after what he had done for me at the 20X, I didn't want to let him down. Sweat burst out of my forehead, which only seconds before had been dry but now was a lawn sprinkler. Drops appeared everywhere, on the mat, the box, the barbell, the kettle bell. A metallic tang hit the back of my throat. Time seemed to be standing still, and now there was no noise, only a bar to lift or a box to jump on and precious air to try to suck into my lungs, as I swung, pressed, and jumped.

The announcer broke the reverie. "One minute to go!" he screamed. Paul screamed, too, but I don't know what he said. I knew I had slowed down, that 120 wasn't close. His words came into focus: he wanted me to grab the bar and pump out seven more presses. What had felt like a mere pillow now felt like deadweight. Seven seemed out of the realm of possibility. If I dropped the bar after lifting it overhead, I was spared the effort of lowering it. But then I would have to lift it from the ground, a time-consuming move. I found a spot in the distance, an exit sign over a door in the ski lodge, and focused on it. One press. Down to my chest. Focus. Breathe. A second press. Down to my chest. Two breaths. Paul screams. The announcer screams. I breathe, try to focus, push. Another. Another . . .

"Three, two, one, TIME!" I drop the bar and collapse in a puddle of my own sweat and spit and try to breathe. Paul is screaming, pounding my back as it heaves, beyond my control. "You did it! You did it! You got a hundred and one reps!" he says, happier for me than I am for myself. I rise to my knees after a minute, one knee after two, the acid subsiding, the breath returning, the sweat still pouring. I stand up, hug Paul, and high-five and fist-bump the other Annex athletes as we file out of the Pit. Paul is by my side, hand on my lower back again, ecstatic. "I knew you could do it," he says.

"Only because of you," I gasp. "Thank you. Thank you."

Paul laughed at me; he had another round to judge and was gone.

We moved immediately into a chute lined with tables filled with cups of water. We had a few minutes before the obstacle run started, so we deconstructed the workout. Turns out I did get my ass kicked by the other Annex members, especially Mickey, who got in 133 reps and barely broke a sweat. Everyone else got in at least 115 reps, which didn't bode well for the run. True, I had done a seven-mile run with Anne, kind of on a lark, about a month before, and was surprised at how easy it felt, despite the fact that I hadn't run much more than two miles at a pop. But we were putting Tabata's principles to the test here: short-duration training can equal long-duration efforts.

I hoped he was right. He'd better be right. These people were strong.

They showed it when the gun went off to send us on

our way. While I was content to lumber along and conserve energy for what lay ahead, my teammates bolted off, energy conservation apparently not an issue. After five hundred yards or so of a course that wound through Camelback's base area and water park, we came to the first obstacle: we were to get from one side of the water park's wave tank to the other, deep end, and haul ourselves up and out on cargo nets. No problem, for me. I put my head down and swam, all awkward with boots and long shorts but feeling more in my element now that gravity's effects had been lessened. I swam, keeping an eye on Anne, a decent swimmer, but I wanted to be sure she could get up the nets. I reached them first (the last time today I would be first over anything), hauled myself out, and reached down to help the others. Here we were, a team.

The others bolted off, down a short, slippery hill toward a series of wooden walls of varying height. We were all thoroughly soaked from the tank, and it had started to rain, turning the dirt trails into rinks of mud and making the obstacles slick. Here's where I can be a good teammate, I thought. I'm a good climber, I'm not afraid of heights, and I can encourage everyone up and over. Some of the Annex ladies had professed to a fear of heights. But from the way they vaulted, pulled, and threw themselves over the barriers, some of them a mere four feet, some as high as fifteen, I started to think that these were the people who thought using epidurals during childbirth was a character flaw. Nobody looked scared. Or winded. Or like they needed a teammate's help.

We ran on, starting to string out over the course, through a long, unlit drainage pipe, ankle-deep in cold water. Along a creek bed, hopping from rock to rock, using the small trees that crowded the banks as hand grips. We ran up some small hills and back down them, climbing over a container box in the middle. Anne wanted to run off with the others, to keep up and then beat them. She never said as much, but I could tell. But she stayed with me as I lumbered along. The farther I fell behind, the more I could feel anger rising in my blood, flowing the same pathways as the lactic acid. Mad that I was falling behind, that I was the weak link. Mad that they were faster than me. Mad that we weren't working together. It was the bad voice, and I told it to shut up.

Soon we headed up a snowcat track that switchbacked across the ski slope. All but the smallest and fastest of the competitors started walking, some with heads held high, some with heads sagging. A race volunteer handed me a sandbag, probably about a 35-pounder, and told me to follow the others up the hill. I did, but I was losing contact. I tried hard, but I knew that at some point we were going to go over the top of the mountain, and I'd need to conserve some energy, because we weren't even halfway there.

Just as I was about to stop to catch my breath, the trail bent to the left and then dipped straight down a ski slope.

The relief I felt was fleeting, for no sooner did my lungs stop searing from the effort of the climb than my quads started to buckle from the exertion of controlling myself and my load on the slick descent. I used one hand to stabilize the bag that lay draped over my shoulder and the other to wave in the air to balance myself. It worked, and after about five minutes I was able to drop the bag, grab a cup of water, and catch up to Anne, who looked at me as if she was, not mad at me, but really, really disappointed.

"How are you doing?" she asked.

I told her I felt pretty good.

"You're not supposed to feel good," she said, smiling but intense, her voice rising the way it does when she really, really means something. "It's a race. It's *supposed* to hurt."

I wish I could say this was the first time I had heard this from her, but when, some fifteen years before, she saw a photo of me crossing the finish line of the 1998 New York City Marathon with my arms spread wide like an airplane and a big smile on my face as the clock flashed 4:13.28, she had simply shook her head and said, "If you were smiling at the finish line, you didn't run hard enough." To prove her point, she showed me a picture of herself taken at the same finish line a few years before, her eyes vacant, her face a death mask of pain, her time forty-five minutes faster than mine. She had told me the same thing at the CRASH-B Sprints, an indoor rowing competition I had scored a Plimptonesque assignment to cover. She watched me race, and when I finished, in a personal-best time for a 2,000-meter row, she shook her head and said, "You could have gone faster. You're too conservative."

The first few times she said this to me, in the early days of our marriage, it pissed me off. I had never run a marathon, and was happy merely to have finished one. And when I had completed the CRASH-Bs 2000, I had lain in a heap on the gym floor for five minutes trying to find the strength to sit up. I certainly felt as if I had gone hard enough. But here was my wife telling me I was a slacker. Had I added another bad voice to the chorus?

But as the marriage went on, and I listened to Anne describe her own workouts, I realized she wasn't telling me anything she didn't tell herself. When she'd come home from a run, I'd ask her how it was. "It was awful," she'd say. "I don't know what's happening. I'm so slow." This was usually said while she had a bag of frozen peas on both knees in an effort to reduce the swelling of her redlined effort. Or "I didn't push hard enough today." Anne had the same desire to always be at the front that I had. But she also had an ability that I didn't have. Even after having three kids in less than two years and holding down a full-time job, Anne could go to state-level triathlons and finish in the top three in her age group. She was hard on herself, and it bore results.

Now all that came rushing back in the rain at Camelback Mountain. "Thanks, coach!" I said, headed back up the slope, wondering un-idle thoughts about marriage and running and running with your spouse. There was no switchback to this trail. It blasted straight up the hill, following a ski lift line. There was no running; at times, there was no walking, the trail so steep we were forced to all-fours to bear-crawl our way up. People from later waves were passing us, and I could tell Anne was getting more and more pissed. But she didn't leave her man behind.

At long last we reached a wide trail that traversed the summit of the mountain. Sweet relief, I thought as we paused at a water station and I shook my legs, hoping to get some blood back into them. I looked across the traverse and saw what must have been five steel barricades, all about chest high. The only way over them was a vault. I'm glad the course photographers seemed to have been scared off by the rain that now fell steadily. After such a long slog up, there was no spring, no vault, left in me, and however I threw myself over the barricades in what must have looked like a halfhearted attempt to hump them, it would not have made a pretty picture. But we got over them. There waiting for us was the rest of Team Annex. They had waited.

But they could smell the barn, and so the descent of the mountain, which for sanity's and ankles' sake should have followed the switchbacks, instead ran right down the fall line, the straightest, steepest, scariest way down. It was now my turn to wait for Anne, whose bad knees and fear of falling (she hates skiing, diving, and mountain biking) forced her to rein herself in. I was only too glad to return the favor, the rest coming as a blessing. We could see the finish line, hear the manic voice of the announcer as he read out finishers' names and hometowns. It will be fun to finish, I thought. Two hours of this stuff is enough.

But we weren't headed to the finish line. Not just yet. The trail I thought headed there instead veered off to a small pond near the base lodge. There were ropes strung from a dock on one side to a dock on the other, suspended about four feet above the water. We were to grab the rope with our hands, lock our ankles around it, and pull ourselves across. Ropes, water, whatever, I thought. I got this. I did. So did Anne. Not so many of the other competitors, who seemed to be freaking out at the thought of getting wet and dropping from the ropes like ripe pears into the murky pond. Feeling smug for the first time all day, I hauled out on the other side and did my best to sound encouraging and help the fallen up onto the dock. I was slow, but I could stay wet.

Finally, finally, finally, we reached the last obstacle: Camelback Beach's Lazy River. Instead of rafts or noodles to ease us down the flume, we were to wade right in and walk through the water, maybe three hundred yards or so. I decided it would be faster to swim, and soon some of my teammates were swimming. Rather than a lazy breast-stroke or crawl down the Lazy River, they took turns doing the far more taxing butterfly. Because, you know, the last two hours weren't hard enough.

But we all came in the same way we started: together. They had waited for me. I'm sure it killed them, but nobody said anything to me.

"Here comes TEAAAAAMM ANNNNNEXXXX!" the finish line announcer screamed like a tattooed Ed McMahon to the six or so people gathered around the finish line. The rain was a major buzzkill, and the party the organizers had promised for the finish line was a bust. I gave my beer ticket to Anne, who pounded down a Bud Lite like it was Gatorade. I stripped off my shoes and socks and let my pruned toes breathe. I sat on a wooden chair under an overhang and watched the rain fall and a few of my teammates suck down beer. I was amazed that with zero specific training for an event like this, save for the Pit, I was able to just jump in and do it. Sure it wasn't fast, but I completed it. CrossFit had prepared me pretty well, I thought, even if I did need to figure out a way to run faster over distance. I was pretty happy. The happiness didn't fade a bit when I remembered what faced me over the next eight days: Murph, and a 3.5-mile ocean swim.

Still, it felt good to sit. It was an hour's drive to get home, and I knew that all the time sitting would only make me stiffer, but I didn't care. I had done well in the Pit, worked hard on the hill, and now could think about a relaxing Saturday night on the couch, the night of cheat day, eating pizza and drinking a bottle of good red wine. The Annex ladies emerged from the bathroom.

Not a trace of mud or fatigue to be seen and their hair looked great. They had to run, they said. They had to get home. There was a school benefit that night. "Bye!" And off they danced.

When we got home, I unfolded myself, slowly, from the car, chased ibuprofen with a beer, took a long, hot shower, and settled into the couch. It was bliss. The next day I was sore as hell, sore all over, too sore to even consider a workout, which is really saying something because when you work a full-time job, the Sunday workout is sacrosanct. It is the way to be sure you get in at least one workout that week. I stretched and used the foam roller, lazily, in front of the TV. On Monday, sufficiently recovered to work out, I lifted easily and did a short (4:56) workout of jump rope and moving a barbell from the ground to over my head. I was surprised at how good it felt, as if my blood vessels and muscles were rusty pipes and the exercise was hot water flushing them out. I took Tuesday off from everything, going so far as to take cabs the mile between Penn Station and my office, despite the beautiful weather. On Wednesday I swam in a pool for thirty minutes, and on Thursday ran some 400s as part of a WOD.

I felt as ready as I was going to be for Murph.

Friday morning was cool and showery. A group of eight of us gathered for the 5:30 WOD, and nobody looked too happy, above and beyond the sheer shittiness of getting up at 5 a.m. to do this to ourselves. (Except for Gephart, a freakishly strong and optimistic guy with a shaved head that glistened when he sweat. He was strapping on a weight vest with the same glee the Hanson Brothers put on the foil.) We had all done Murph before, and knew what was ahead of us. It was a flat-out beatdown. But unlike most of the other Hero WODs, we now had a two-degrees-of-separation relationship with the man for whom the workout was named. Before we began, I told the guys what Mark Divine and Instructor Brad, the guy with the David Byrne glasses, had told us at the 20X, about how they knew Murph, and how his sacrifice—exposing himself to certain death in order to save his comrades—was an act of valor few people can conceive of. This was why the WOD was almost a sacrament to these guys. And why Divine would accept nothing less than everything an athlete had when he was doing Murph. "I'm not saying I'll beat any of you guys," I told the group. "I'll probably be last. But I will be going as hard as I can."

The mood in the room changed. Everyone stood a little taller. Those of us doing the WOD with the additional load of a twenty-pound weight vest—body armor—cinched the straps a little bit tighter. We all bumped fists before the clock started, something we never do, and gave each other a nod.

Running a mile with a weight vest on, and trying to do it with some semblance of speed, is probably the hardest thing I've done at CrossFit. Every time I do it, I'm reminded of the saying a bicycle company engineer once told me when I asked why light gear was so expensive: "Light, strong, cheap. Pick two." The CrossFit equivalent is light, strong, and fast. CrossFit had made me strong, and lighter when measured by body fat. But I was by no means faster, especially right now. I was DFL in the run, behind even notorious plodder Big Man Jerry, who liked running as much as he liked pull-ups.

It didn't matter. I was putting out, as best I could. I used a strap to help with the pull-ups, but I chipped away, 10 at a time, followed by 20 push-ups and 30 air squats. Ten cycles of that. Steve Gephart was miles ahead of me, as was Leo, as they executed butterfly pull-ups a gymnast would envy. For my part, I did the 30 squats unbroken each time, and did the 20 push-ups as hand release, harder than normal push-ups, but like at the 20X, a nod to the fact that I was using a band on the pull-ups. By the time I was on my seventh set, Gephart and Leo were out the door, running their miles as Jerry and I kept at it. The floor was an ocean of commingled sweat. The vest dug into my shoulders and sides. Now the others were finished, slapping hands and talking about how much it sucked.

A year ago, I would have been pissed off. At them, and at myself. Now, I was psyched for them, happy they could go so fast. And proud of myself for not stopping.

Finally, I was running the last mile. Running might be kind of a strong word to describe my determined plod.

I was hell-bent on not walking, not one step, even on the annoyingly slight grade up to the railroad bridge, then the slight descent to the sign at Passaic River Park, our half-mile marker, the turnaround point. I slapped the sign and turned around. Five more minutes or so to go. I went back up the rise, under the train tracks and had, at last, a view of River Road as it fell away home, to the Annex. I saw a couple of other guys ahead of me in the distance, but I also saw a lone figure on the other side of the road, running toward me. I figured it was someone out for a run, not one of the Annex guys.

But then the figure got closer. It was Gephart, running back up the road. "Dude, you're nuts," I huffed when he got within range. "You need more PT?"

"No, man. I came out to help you back in." Gephart stopped and pivoted, taking up a position on my left shoulder, matching my pace exactly and talking, an easy, non-stop rap designed to take my mind off the effort and the pain of the final six hundred yards or so. No hand on the back, like Paul, but it was just as welcome, and effective, and made my eyes well with tears. As we got closer to the Annex, the guys who had already finished came out and yelled at me to bring it in. Usually, given the time constraints we all face in the morning, the unspoken rule is that you can leave as soon as you're done in order to help get the kids out the door or catch the train. But not today. They waited and yelled until I brought it all the way in, sixty-five minutes, dead last but a personal record. Then we took a picture. In it, we're all smiling. We look tired, and our T-shirts and hair are drenched. But we look happy. Honestly, openly happy at what we were just able to do.

We got up early Saturday to fly to St. John, and each movement I made that day required a supreme effort of will and produced a flood of regret. "What the fuck was I thinking, scheduling all this stuff so close together?" I said to Anne as I shifted in the narrow airplane seat, trying to find a comfortable position. She had done Murph the day before, too, at a later class, after swimming three thousand yards. She wasn't sore. Sleepy, but not sore. Holding a newspaper at arm's length to read produced spasms and cramps in my arms. Picking luggage off the carousel at the airport in St. Thomas was agony. It wasn't that I was sore as much as that my muscles felt completely and utterly depleted, which made movement almost impossible. Not even the warm air and sunshine of St. John, my favorite place on earth, made me feel better. My walk up and down the stairs that led to our hotel room must have looked like physical sketch comedy.

We came to St. John every Memorial Day weekend to join in the Beach-to-Beach Power Swim, a fund-raiser for the national park that comprises about 90 percent of the island. Its presence is the reason the island is so special—a relatively undeveloped speck in the Caribbean, with no airport or deepwater port to allow cruise ship visits, which unleash hordes on neighboring St. Croix and St. Thomas. The swim itself is a rarity in open-water races, a point-to-point jaunt starting at Maho Bay and headed south along the island's west shore. If you want to swim about one mile, you can stop at Cinnamon Bay; if you want to swim about 2.25 miles, you can stop at Trunk Bay. And if you want to go 3.5 miles, you get out at Hawks Nest Beach.

This year, the kids were going to join us. We had made their participation in the trip provisional on the fact that they would all do the one-mile swim; they could use fins if they wanted to, as would I. I wanted them to know they could swim this far, to feel comfortable in the water and to see its beauties. Catherine and Christine, eleven-year-old identical twins, were regulars on our summer pool's swim team. They could handle a mile easily if they just stopped talking and swam. Luke, thirteen, could also handle it, but was more likely to get nervous in the deep water we were going to traverse. The race was very well organized, with tons of kayakers and powerboats along the route, which was marked by giant orange buoys. The plan was for me and Anne to buddy-swim the three of them to Cinnamon, make sure they got out okay, then the two of us would continue on to Hawks Nest.

That was the plan. And as we stood ankle-deep in the soft warm water at Maho, the sun just peaking over the hills behind us and schools of tiny fish bumping against our feet, I knew with certainty that the plan would work. I knew the kids would be fine, even if they didn't know it at that moment. I knew that I'd loosen up and enjoy the swim, and that I was fit enough to do this, to finish the triple crown, and to wear my participant T-shirts with pride.

Most of the people I know, especially very fit ones, are paralyzed by water in general and swimming in particular. It's both understandable and lamentable. Understandable because most adults don't spend enough time in the water to develop the degree of comfort they need to push their limits the way they can on dry land. Put too much weight on a bar and fail at an overhead squat and all you have to do is bail out by dropping the bar. Get a cramp while running a marathon and you can sit on the curb and massage it away. But swallow a bunch of seawater a mile from shore and you need to be able to tread water until you are able to cough it back up and get your shit together. That's a skill that takes some practice. The key is training yourself to not panic. One of the reasons more than 90 percent of deaths that occur during triathlons happen during swims, I'm convinced, is that people panic when they hit the water because they're just not comfortable enough in it, and the panic leads to heart attacks. Plus, when you enter a pond or the ocean, you're entering a wilderness. Who knows what lurks in that murky water? That freaks out people. I choose not to think about it. I feel sorry for them because I have known a peace and joy in the water that I find hard to duplicate while dry. I wish everyone could experience it.

My buoyancy helps. Part of the reason I like the water is that the spare tire that has long held me back on land like some sort of anchor actually works to my advantage by affording me a degree of floatiness that other, leaner athletes lack. Olympic swimmers have an average body fat percentage (6–12 percent for men) that's 4 percentage points higher than distance runners (2–8). Whether the extra bit of subdermal fat—and let's be clear here, nobody would call Michael Phelps fat—helps the person swim or whether the relatively cool water in which they spend so much training time holds back fat depletion is still up for debate, but I can tell you for sure that my friend Loren, an All-American runner, is an ace thrasher in the pool, and Chris, who can routinely ride and run me into the ground, takes an awfully long time to complete the swimming leg of a triathlon.

There's another dirty little secret at play here. Most people approach swimming as if it were running or cycling, and think that the key to getting faster is to swim more. But their strokes suck. When they swim more, all they do is reinforce bad form and their muscles remember doing something wrong. Better to approach it as if it were a golf swing, or a power snatch. Get some coaching, learn and reinforce good form, and all of a sudden you'll feel more comfortable because you're breathing easier, so you spend more time in the water, get more comfortable . . . and the circle completes itself.

Anne is the perfect example of this. When we met, in 1996, she was uncomfortable even putting her face under a shower stream. She couldn't swim from one end of a pool to another without panicking. But after attending a few clinics and camps, and swimming twice a week without fail with a triathlon club at the Summit, New Jersey, YMCA, she's now a respectable and fearless swimmer. And she beat me in a 5K swim once.

One more thing: Think about how kids play in the water. They don't swim laps. They play sharks-and-minnows and dive to the bottom of the pool and see who can hold their breath the longest and who can make the biggest splash off the diving board. They're comfortable because they're playing. They develop confidence through play.

So the thought of a swim, one in which I could use fins, didn't faze me in the least. I was with my family and would have to make sure everyone was okay, to be the sheepdog of the group, but that was fine with me. A little backing and forthing, more yards? No worries. I got this. I was sore, but I was still strong. And I was in the ocean.

Remember cartoons from the hippie days, the ones where all the animals and races live together in peace and harmony and all the colors are superbright and the rays of the sun strong and helpful and everyone digs each other in a Technicolor kind of way and the music is groovy and everything is good and happy? That's what this swim was like. At least, that's what my memories of it are. I've done enough long swims to know that I was probably sore and chafed and really thirsty by the time I finished, but to be in eighty feet of clear, Caribbean water, doing something I love, with the people I love, and watching my kids overcome their nerves and not just thrive but succeed— Christine won her age group and got a glass medal. Catherine finished second.

Or maybe it was swimming along and seeing turtles and rays below us, and navigating our route by the lush peaks on nearby St. Thomas.

I know for a fact that had the kids not been there, I would have tried to race, and that would have been a disaster because I didn't have enough left in the tank for a really hard effort. I had finished third in my age group in this race the previous two years, and I would have wanted to do that, or better, again. I would have been plagued with thoughts of how, in my late twenties and early thirties, I could go to an open-water swim race and reasonably expect to finish in the top five.

Not this time. Instead, I sidestroked and breaststroked

and dog-paddled, stopping every once in a while to make sure the kids were okay with a shaka, our agreed-upon symbol for things being good. They'd pop their heads up like seals every once in a while and yell, "Turtle!" and we'd all dive down to follow the thing as it glided along. Sometimes they'd float on their backs like otters, flutter-kicking to keep forward progress while giving their arms a break. We stopped once to form a circle in the water, everybody checking on everybody else.

When the kids got out at the one-mile point, Anne and I kept on. She told me to go ahead, not to wait for her, but after what she did for me at Camelback, I owed her and told her I'd stay with her. "No, you're using fins," she said. "You're way faster. Go ahead."

And so I did, letting the steady swell from the north push me along, stopping to talk to the dudes in the small boats handing out bottles of fresh water, even floating on my back to give my arms a break and take in the sky. It was amazing.

It was amazing because I could do it. And I could do it because I was fit. Everything I had been able to achieve in the last nine days was possible because of all those moments lying on the stinky plastic turf at the Annex, staring at the ceiling, catching my breath. I was never alone when I was there. The other guys were there, but so was my mother, standing behind my father, telling me she'd drive me to the race, and that of course I could ride thirty-two miles. I was never alone over the last nine days. In fact, the efforts I thought were solo were anything but. I was carried along by the efforts of other people, and of their connection to each other. That's why I had told Mark Divine that love was the answer. That's what I meant.

We had a big meal that night, with lots of good beer from the local brewery. The next day we played tennis and snorkeled.

There was no box on St. John, but we didn't miss it. We had our fitness.

We had our answer.

# Epilogue

## April 12, 2014

Anne and I did the 6 a.m. class today. There were only four of us. Nola, the coach, had us do a ton of mobility work to start and a nice long warm-up, which felt really good after the hard-lifting WOD I had put myself through last night. The three guys finishing up the early class looked like they were working hard, but nobody seemed like they were going to die. Jeff, whom I hadn't seen in a while, looked as if he had been lifting a lot—his arms were big. I told him so, and got a shy, appreciative smile in return.

We ran 400s in the gloaming just before dawn, the steam rising from our sweaty heads as we ran back and forth across the parking lot. We came inside and did snatches and overhead walking lunges and double unders, completed, as usual, to the background duet of the humming of the spinning ropes and the by-now ritual chant of "FUCCCCKKKK!!" from those of us inadvertently whipping ourselves with them. The whole thing was over in, for me, 15 minutes and 24 seconds. I was last. Anne ran me into the ground, as did Mark and Tim. I lifted more in the snatches, but after all this time, 400s still kill me.

When it was over, I sat on a wooden box and caught my breath. After running 400s, it took a while. That's when I noticed something: I was looking at the wall, not the ceiling. The workout was hard, but rather than leaving me prostrate on the floor, I was able to catch my breath while sitting on a box; I didn't need to collapse in a heaving, sweaty heap.

Nor did I beat myself into submission for coming in last. I had done my best. I wish I had run faster. I've been wishing that my entire life. But I ran as hard as I could, hard enough to get a thumbs-up from two guys walking down the street who had stumbled onto our predawn ritual. Not that affirmation from two total strangers meant all that much. But the fact that I smiled and waved in response to their small gesture of support signaled to me that I had crossed a watershed. I was running with people, measuring myself against them, but still finding joy in the movement and the freedom that came with it. I had found a pleasure and a meaning that had nothing to do with how I compared against other people. I was doing it because I could.

A lot has changed since I began my experiment to Embrace the Suck. My body, for one. My weight has stayed pretty much the same as it was since I ended the Paleo Challenge at CrossFit Morristown. But I now have a physique the fat kid in the Husky Boy department never dreamed possible. My pants are looser and shirts and jackets are all tighter. I like having a big back, and I like seeing veins in my arms and hands. And I like not feeling a jiggle around my belt when I run to catch a train.

There are lots of smaller, subtler changes, too. A couple of months ago, while shopping in a Walgreen's with Christine, we found ourselves trapped in a narrow aisle. We backed up blindly to escape a crush of shopping carts coming at us from either end of the aisle. I stumbled over a stepladder, but rather than falling flat on my ass, I was able to catch my balance and stay upright. When I wondered aloud at my minor act of body control brilliance, Christine looked at me and said, simply, "CrossFit." She was right: I had a linkage between the different parts of my body that had never existed before. I can now sprint to catch a train and actually make it. And running up the stairs at Penn Station after a workout no longer leaves me winded.

My knowledge of diet and my appreciation for the effect it can have on that physique is much deeper than it ever was, even if I won't fully embrace the fire breathers' diet. Perhaps it's lame, but I feel that there's room in my life for both CrossFit and Peanut M&Ms, and although the two may not be complementary, they are not mutually exclusive, at least not to me.

Perhaps that explains why certain moves continue to elude me, despite my best efforts. I still don't have a muscle-up, and my kip still sucks. Would they come to me if I dropped another twenty pounds? Maybe. Do I lose sleep over the fact that I can't do a muscle-up? Only when someone like Joe tells me he did fifty of them on a recent Saturday morning, as a way to mark his fiftieth birthday.

Some things haven't changed. Anne still calls me every morning after the 8:45 WOD to tell me how she did and grouse about how sucky running is. Lifting continues to be my favorite part of the WODs. Mickey started teaching a Saturday morning Olympic lifting class, which I go to as often as I can to have the sensei critique my form. My one-rep maxes have gone up in all of the four basic lifts thanks to Mick's help, and to my own diligence.

Running continues to suck for me, too, but I continue to do it, a boat against the current.

What I no longer do is wonder whether I belong, at CrossFit or anyplace else. Not at work, not at home, not at the head of a family. It's not about how I compare to the rest of the world. It's about showing up and doing your best and not giving up on a promise. There's a lesson to be learned in embracing the suck. But there's a greater lesson to be learned in embracing it all. The stronger your arms, the tighter your embrace.

What makes me think I can do this?

I do.

# Afterword

A lot has happened since the first edition of *Embrace the Suck* was published in December 2014. CrossFit continues to grow, the Annex moved into a vast new space, and the exigencies of life have driven some changes in my approach to fitness.

CrossFit marches on. There are now more than 13,000 affiliated gyms around the world, about half of them in the

United States. I've been to boxes in places ranging from Toronto to Grand Cayman to Paris, and the fervor with which people attack "le WODs" is the same, regardless of the continent. The CrossFit Games are now a mainstay of summer TV viewing on ESPN, Crossfit has 840,000 followers on Twitter alone, and Reebok/CrossFit continues to build shiny new boxes around the world.

Sometimes I wonder if, in its growth, CrossFit hasn't lost something that was a big part of its appeal: an underground, garagiste feeling that this was something for a unique few, not made for everyone. I mentioned it one morning at the Annex, and Leo promptly reminded me of how nice it was to have a place to work out in January, when the temperature in my garage was 14 degrees. And if more people want to be able to do pull-ups, then run a mile, that's a good thing.

And you can't argue with results. I continue to appreciate with amazement the way CrossFit has changed the bodies and attitudes of people who walk through the door of the Annex. Stay-at-home moms and middle-aged executives alike continue to get their asses kicked during the on-ramp instructional sessions, and they continue to come back for more. Some people have moved on, of course. A bunch of the women who ran the Civilian Military Combine trained for and ran the 2016 New York City Marathon. They stopped coming to the Annex while they trained, and most of them never came back, favoring a combination of running and Barre Method to maintain their fitness. Duignan, hobbled by injuries, switched to a more cardio-intensive regimen called Orange Theory. When I see him on the train into New York City, he sheepishly swears he'll be back at the Annex someday.

My regular 5:30 a.m. group faded, resurged, and faded again. Rutter moved to England, Gerry decided to focus on tossing the shot put at master's track meets and became a national age-group champion. Steve and Nola moved to Tennessee. Joe and Leo keep on, but not as often, although always with the same manic intensity, knee injuries and impending triathlons posing no barrier.

A new group emerged at the Annex after Mickey moved the facility to a huge new space that includes a 50-yard-long stretch of indoor Astroturf, a yoga studio, and a pitching mound, where he trains athletes like the 2016 American League Cy Young Award winner, Rick Porcello. The new space allowed Mickey to expand his CrossFit gear as well as his programming. The result was the rise of a competitors' group, true fire-breathers who meet every day at 7:30 to do a special workout, because for these guys and girls, the regular WODs aren't hard enough. They tend to be younger, in their twenties, and add a new level of intensity, humor, and performance to the Annex crowd, even if their taste in music can seem perplexing to us silverbacks.

They're not all, kids, though. One of their members is Jamie Cutler, a former Marine now in his late forties.

# Afterword

When Jamie walked into the Annex, he was huge from weight lifting, but had zero flexibility and no endurance. He could throw around weight, but that was about it. Now, two years of chipping away later, he's one of the premier examples of the alchemy that can occur when perseverance and sheer stubbornness are combined with the CrossFit protocol.

I say he's one of the premier examples, but he's not the premier example. I'm biased of course, but that title belongs to Anne, who has so completely embraced CrossFit that, with the exception of swimming twice a week and occasional forays to the track, has given up all other fitness pursuits. At 8 each evening, she begins checking her phone to see if the next day's workout has been posted on the Annex website. And despite having her own business to run—or perhaps because of it—she does an amazing job of organizing her schedule so she can remain a regular at the 8:45 a.m. WOD. She still calls me right after the WOD to discuss the results.

And the results are amazing. Anne's body has been utterly transformed from that of a lithe runner to that of a person who can throw around Olympic weights with ease and abandon. She's always had a big engine, but now any WOD that requires leg strength or overhead strength, Anne crushes. I can't keep up with her. She looks better in tights at age fifty than she did at thirty.

As for me, CrossFit remains an important part of a

complicated life, but circumstances have forced me to put other things first. That start-up I was running, the one with the four demanding bosses who led me to feel the need to toughen up mentally, it went the way of most start-ups just before the first edition was published and I found myself out of a job.

Unemployment can be a boon for personal fitness. All of a sudden you have plenty of time on your hands to go to the box, do the WOD, and stay around afterward to work on skills like pull-ups or double unders. If you're forced to economize, you eat out less, which makes maintaining or losing weight easier.

And all the lessons I learned at the box—chip away, one rep at a time, things take time, hard work brings results, form matters—came into play at one time or another while I looked for a job and worked as a consultant on a variety of publishing projects. They became mantras that helped me to cope with the frustrations and indignities of the job search, and allowed for victory cries to be crowed when work came through.

And it did. At this writing, I'm the editorial director of a company that publishes websites and magazines for hobbyists. About the time I got the job, I sustained my first CrossFit-induced injury, a pulled lower back muscle that exploded as I reached the bottom of a back squat. I could barely move for a week, and when I could, I became unwilling to commit to the full range of motion needed for a proper workout. Then I had three teeth pulled and a bunch of skin cancers removed. It became a real effort to work out.

When I could no longer fit into my favorite pair of jeans, I shook it off. But it's hard to find the level of intensity I once had. That's going into my work, and my family. Luke, Catherine, and Christine are teenagers now and will be leaving for the world beyond Chatham in three short years. I don't want to miss anything, so I don't go to bed early to rise for the 5:30 a.m. WOD.

My work requires a lot of travel, though, which means I've become familiar with boxes in Cincinnati and Fort Collins, Colorado. I drop in, I do the WOD, but I garner attention mostly for being the oldest person at the box; CrossFit remains primarily a young person's pursuit, and at fifty-three, almost everyone looks young to me. I also do a lot of hotel gym and hotel room workouts: push-ups, sit-ups, and squats that taken together maintain some form of fitness. But I won't be joining the 7:30 a.m. fire-breathers at the Annex any time soon. I'm lucky to get to the Annex three times a week now, usually with Anne, who finishes way ahead of me, then graciously brings me a towel and lets me have a swig from her Poland Spring bottle.

But still, after a lifetime of embracing the suck, I know how to put out, and I know why I should put out. Yesterday I shuffled twelve miles around Paris in a frigid rain, thinking as I lost the feeling in my hands and nose that there was a lot of suck to embrace in this particular work-out. And this morning I ran sprints for half an hour on the quays along the Left Bank of the Seine, the sun rising behind Notre Dame before being chased away by low scudding clouds that brought more rain, rain that chased me to the cafe where I write this.

Not much that sucks there. But like my life, so much to embrace.

# Acknowledgments

Writers typically wait until the very end of their book's acknowledgments section to thank their families, who bear the brunt of the insanity that comes from the process of writing. This is absurdly backward. So allow me to start by thanking my wife, Anne Thompson, and our children, Luke, Catherine, and Christine, for putting up with me while I wrote this book. I was physically absent most weekends for a few months while I finished the book, and even when I was around I wasn't fully present, the act of writing being something that's hard to put down just because you're trying to have a nice family dinner or watch a basketball game. Plus, how many nights did I fall asleep on the couch or pull myself away from you all so I could get enough sleep before the early WOD? So to them I say: Thank you for your patience, your generosity, and your love. It is always the answer.

Anybody who writes a fitness memoir owes a debt to those who have written on the topic before him. Specifically, I want to thank Bill Strickland and Bill McKibben, whose *Ten Points* and *Long Distance*, respectively, influenced how I came to think about writing, sports, and sports writing.

I'd also like to thank the teachers, editors, and colleagues who helped me learn the craft of reporting, editing, and writing over the years: Sister Henrietta, ND; William Collins; John Marcham; Keith Johnson; Chris Dornan; Jack Krieger; Joe Junod; Susan Fraker; David Bauer; David Willey; Jon Dorn; Peter Flax; Jay Heinrichs; Loren Mooney; Nancy Nasworthy; Andrea Barbalich; and Paul Cody.

At CrossFit Annex, in Chatham, New Jersey, a thanks for the friendship and encouragement go to Nola Gephart, Steve Gephart, Gerry Donini, Leo Paytas, Dave Rutter, Joe Berkery, John LeRoy, Tommy Fuccello, Stefan Weber, Muffie Roarke, John Paone, Matt Spiegel, Crystal Paone, Beth DeCicco, Matt DeCicco, Edwin Rambusch, Martin Rambusch, Chris Duignan, and Lisa Coleman. Special thanks to Mickey Brueckner for being such a good coach and even more so for building such a strong and special community within his place of business. Some businesses change lives for the better; the Annex is one of them.

At CrossFit Morristown (now Guerrilla Fitness), thanks to Karianne Dickson, Leo Munoz, and Mike DelaTorre for their enthusiasm and generosity in teaching me the fundamentals of CrossFit. Thanks also to Greg Glassman for thinking up this stuff and making it open source, and to Tony Budding for explaining things so clearly.

At HarperWave, I owe a huge debt of gratitude to my editor, Karen Rinaldi, who entertained the idea of a book about CrossFit way back when, before CrossFit had entered the mainstream, and who pushed me to places I didn't want to go in order to tell this story completely. Karen is a fine editor, a bad-ass water woman, and an even better psychologist, who pulled much of this book from under the shale ledges in my psyche, and for that I will always be grateful. Also, thanks to the entire HarperWave team, especially Jake Zebede, Heather Drucker, Tom Hopke Jr., and the countless others who helped get this book into the light of day.

After almost fifty years of doing this stuff, the list of people who have shared the pain and the fun of the pursuit might be incomplete, but I need to acknowledge the following people for sharing the pleasure and the pain of the workouts and the discovery. John Griffin, Bill Elberry,

## Acknowledgments

Michael Green, Coach John Normant, Charles Lyons, Matthew Stewart, Christine Rossiter, Shelly Matheney, Kevin Valleley, Steve Somogy, Phil "The Hammer" Iorio, Francesca Crannell, Trish Pagliarulo, Seth Cohen, Craig Schiffer, Mike Fabajanic, Carl Sangree, Chris Lambiase, Terry Londeree, and Stefan Weber.

I also need to thank United Airlines and New Jersey Transit for providing environments surprisingly conducive to writing if not to comfort, and to the family at Drip Coffee in Madison, New Jersey, for their care for and support of freeloading writers who pay $4.28 for a double espresso then take up space for two hours or more. Thanks also to Starbucks the world over for doing the same thing.

And finally, thanks to my siblings—Maryellen, Bob, Dick, Tim, and Paul—and siblings-in-law—Beth and Michael—who taught me how to read and write, and how to skate, ride, run, and hit. We don't say it to each other enough, but we should: Love is the answer.

# About the Author

STEPHEN MADDEN is the chief content officer for the enthusiast publisher F+W Media. He was the founding editor of *Outdoor Explorer*, as well as the websites Sports on Earth and Fitbie. Madden has held various staff positions at *Sports Illustrated*, *Fortune*, and *Bicycling*, where under his editorship the magazine won two National Magazine Awards. His writing has appeared in more than twenty-five publications and websites.